Take Off Your Party Dress

Take Off Your Party Dress

WHEN LIFE'S TOO BUSY FOR BREAST CANCER

Dina Rabinovitch

POCKET
BOOKS

LONDON • SYDNEY • NEW YORK • TORONTO

First published in Great Britain by Pocket Books, 2007
An imprint of Simon & Schuster UK Ltd
A CBS COMPANY

1 3 5 7 9 10 8 6 4 2

Simon & Schuster UK Ltd
Africa House
64–78 Kingsway
London WC2B 6AH

www.simonsays.co.uk

Simon & Schuster Australia
Sydney

A CIP catalogue record for this book
is available from the British Library

ISBN 13: 978-1-4165-2788-6
ISBN 10: 1-4165-2788-5

Typeset by M Rules
Printed and bound in Great Britain by
Cox & Wyman Ltd, Reading, Berks

For Anthony

Contents

Acknowledgements

First and foremost, the doctors. I've never had my own team of anything before, and thank you for letting me do this without demurring: Mr Muhamed Al-Dubaisi, Dr Peter Ostler and Dr Glenda Kaplan.

Thank you to my alternative community at the *Guardian* including Matt Seaton, Kath Viner, Sarah Crown, Jane Glentworth, Becky Gardiner, Emily Wilson, the two Pauls and all the subeditors who cheered me on: every single one of your messages was a boon and a comfort. Above all, Ian Katz, who swore eternal devotion to my column, and who even, I believe, answered a good three of my emails. To Oliver and Joanna, you two understand just how much those downloads meant. Thank you to the people who came out of the blue, Philip Pullman, Cherie Booth-Blair, Lucy Allen, Kasia Boddy, Sue Shields, all of you scattering gifts, and thank you to that other community of children's writers – with all your wisdom and insights I don't think even you realize how much comfort you brought, especially Adèle Geras and HoTA (Husband of The Adèle) for keeping in touch throughout. There are too many of you to name, but thank you to all the friends who took this road with me, thank you Myrna, Elly, Chany, Tatiana and Milan, and most especially the thousands who responded to my *Guardian* columns and to my blog appeal to raise money for cancer research: we are the tents of Jacob. And thank you Tracy and Andrew, for running with this all the way, and of course, Kerri. I couldn't have crossed the finishing line without you, Michala.

There are the drugs, there are all the cures, but finally, you are the beats of my heart: Anthony, Sara-Jenny, Marganit, Nina, Elon, Max, Laura, Chloë and Theo.

Prologue

'*L*ook, Daddy, look! Quick, Daddy, quick. Look, see, it's flat!' My son Elon is giving a perfect rendition of old-fashioned reading-primer-speak, brought bang up to date with its gritty modern subject matter. Pulling at the towel I've wrapped around myself as I come out of the shower, he's pointing urgently at my breast. Or rather, the place where my breast used to be.

For the first few days after I returned home from hospital, when Elon saw me undressed in the bathroom he stared at the front of me, a startled expression crossing his face. But it was a momentary thing, a second's surprise, before he shifted into some other gear. He made no comment; he didn't seem troubled during the course of his day. This morning, though, he has found the words to express the thought that's been brewing, and it's making him laugh, this comically skewed version of motherhood.

My husband Anthony and I looked hard for a house with room for all the children: at the time, it was four of his and three of mine. We inspected only five- or six-bedroom properties, which narrowed the search considerably. And then we found this home: six bedrooms but, unbelievably, five with their own bathrooms attached.

We moved into the house the morning of the day we married. I came with my three daughters, Sara-Jenny, Marganit and Nina, the girls carrying their pillows on their heads as we entered the new place.

'Quick, you must go straight upstairs.' Myrna, Anthony's mother, met us at the door and rushed us away, petrified that we'd curse the day by running into the other members of this union – Anthony and his four children, Max, Laura, Chloë and Theo – draped on chairs in the kitchen at the back of the house. At 1 p.m. that day we broke the glass under the chuppah, the Jewish marriage canopy, in our conservatory looking out on to the garden. That very night our lives carried on their new rhythms, with some of the children settling down in their rooms while the rest left, to sleep in their other parent's home.

Guests have gathered other times in that conservatory since. But though it's the parties that look out of the photographs, it's the bathrooms, never once photographed, and three of them not much bigger than the children's pencil cases actually, that I bless to this day.

When you're moving an assortment of children of both genders into a living arrangement not of their own choosing, it pays a certain respect to the lines being redrawn to be able to offer the children personal spaces; to say, yes, we are all in this together, but we understand your separatenesses.

Anthony and I, though, have a bathroom with two doors, one to the bedroom and one leading out to the hallway and the rest of the house. Ours is not a private space. Anthony bolts doors but I tend to treat the children like wall tiles, made immune to modesty from the blatantness of hospital childbirths and years of insistent toddlers, and carrying on, often, as if nobody else is in the bathroom, though the place is heavy with small folk. Necessary while children are young, it's a practice which, I discover, survives mastectomy.

But there is also conviction. I think it's better if the children see the scar than if they sense me hiding it and start visualizing what unique grotesquerie I could be masking beneath layers of clothing. I'm sorry, for that reason, that my older daughters no longer barge in on me, because they'd be horrified if I tried to take them aside deliberately to show them what a mastectomy scar looks like.

Elon, anyhow, thinks it's hilarious. This is probably the third or fourth time since my return from hospital that he has caught me undressed.

'I can't see your breast, Mummy,' my little boy says, and, so far from being traumatized, he's chuckling as he points to my right side, where a deep-red lateral scar zigzags from my heart over to my underarm. I remember what the child-psychology books say about answering children's questions about sex: just answer exactly what your child asks, no more, no less. The same rules, I figure, apply here. I have only been able to face looking at myself in the mirror a couple of times since the operation, but this is fine, this is my forte, bringing up fully realized small children, and I'm sitting on the edge of the bath now quite calmly to chat to my youngest.

'Yes,' I say, 'Mummy's skin is covered with cream. It's all white, isn't it?' I have coated the area with lashings of Nivea, in fact, because a nurse tells me its fluffy, whipped-cream texture is good for healing wounds.

'But it's flat, Mummy, why is it flat?'

'It's flat,' I explain, 'because the surgeon took away the bump that was making Mummy ill.'

After the silent, mystified gazes of my first days home, my three-year-old now has a loaded arsenal of questions. 'But how did he do that, Mummy, how did he make it flat?' Elon carries on asking in real wonderment.

'It's flat because the doctor made it flat,' I snap, simultaneously losing both my grip and my not-so-deeply-instilled-after-all good child-rearing practices.

1. Not a Virus, Then

The consultant breast surgeon's name is Mr Al-Dubaisi, and he sees me on Monday evening at the small two-storey hospital, the Garden Clinic, in Hendon, a part of London so little regarded it can't even claim a branch of Starbucks, but where I've lived most of my life.

I like Mr Al-Dubaisi from the moment I meet him. I think I cracked some joke, and he laughed. I can't remember what was funny now, but I remember it was a genuine, throaty chuckle he gave.

He opens a tobacco-coloured paper folder which carries my name on a printed-out label. He pulls over a pristine white sheet of paper from an impeccably stacked pile on the corner of his desk, and takes up a fountain pen, his surgeon's fingers according time to these neat rites. 'When did you first find the lump?' he asks.

When I reply, 'Uh, quite a long time ago, probably when I was pregnant, actually,' he looks up from his sheet of paper.

'Oh, how old's the baby?' He smiles pleasantly.

'He's turning three in a couple of months,' I answer.

He glances up, considering, before moving on. Later, when I say, 'I should have come earlier, shouldn't I?' childlike, seeking dispensation, he offers it instantly.

'We don't talk about what's already happened, no, no, no, it's closed.' His delivery is clipped, precise, like Hercule Poirot.

Then he says, 'I have to ask you something, and you must answer me very, very honestly, Dina.' I freeze. Here it comes. I know what this is, how will I deal with it? He's going to ask me if I mind that he's an Arab. 'Dina,' gently prods this soft, courteous man. 'If it becomes necessary, would it be very inconvenient for you to come and see me at my clinic in Bushey?'

Mr Al-Dubaisi's finely mannered conduct of medical rituals will become a feature of my life. He calls in a chaperone before he gives me a physical examination. He sends me to undress, just my top half, behind orange-patterned curtains in the corner of the room. I can hear him, pacing the room, edgy. I feel he is concerned not to give me a second's extra anxiety, to diagnose a benign lump as soon as possible. The instant the nurse comes through the door, he bursts back through the curtain, energetic, poised for action.

Then he stops still. 'I can see it,' he says, straight away. 'It's large.' His face, which is a warm beige colour, looks momentarily grey. This is not feigned. He doesn't know me at all, this man, but he cares this much.

∾

People have different reactions when you tell them you have breast cancer, and it depends what generation they are from. You see, for the ones like me, late thirties, early forties, it's just beginning to dawn on us that we're the target group now. The sixth series of *Sex and the City*, that tale of four women friends whose gossip became our small talk for the duration of the programmes, was plotted around Samantha's breast cancer. Samantha's hair came out in her boyfriend's fist while they made love, and he lost his erection. Samantha raged at the doctor who told her it was her sex-loaded, pregnancy-free existence that was to blame. 'I'm going to find a woman doctor,' she yelled, 'who knows what she's talking about.'

For children the same age as mine – teenage and younger – it's an illness they are also newly hearing about, in a way it just wasn't part of our lives when we were their age. They know Kylie Minogue, the girl we met as Charlene from the Australian TV soap *Neighbours*, but who they think of only as a pop star, has breast cancer. I watched *Neighbours* every day, collapsed on the couch when I came back from work, while pregnant with my eldest daughter; so much so that the newborn Sara-Jenny recognized the *Neighbours* theme tune when she came out of my womb. Now Charlene's a megastar, and has breast cancer too.

To our burgeoning adolescents it means living with the fact that for about a year and more of their supercharged teen lives, their mothers will be ill. 'I don't want you to change, Mum,' Nina, my ten-year-old says. 'I don't want you to be tired; I don't want you to lose your hair,' she adds, fiercely.

But for the older generation, for people the same age

as my parents, in their seventies now, hearing about our breast cancer is a death knell before our time.

It's an illness older women expect to happen to them, if anyone. Breast cancer screening is given to the over-fifties, routinely. But now breast cancer figures worldwide are running at one in nine women: the highest rates are in the Netherlands and the United States, the lowest in Haiti and the Gambia. It is by far the most common cancer in women.

∽

'But Dina, you read. How could you not know?' asks my mother's old friend, sitting down, hard, on the bench in our hallway.

So here's what I, LSE and University of East Anglia-educated, consumer of two serious newspapers a day, knew. I knew, and so was able to tell my Cambridge-top-of-his-year, multiple-books-a-day husband, with quite impatient certainty, that women like me, who had their first children in their twenties and, what's more – and this was the clincher – breast-fed those babies for well over a year each, women like me don't get breast cancer.

FACT: Having children before the age of twenty or even thirty is protective against breast cancer.
FACT: The longer the period of breast-feeding, the lower the risk of breast cancer for the mother.
(*New England Journal of Medicine*, 1993 and Chris J., 'Women who Breastfeed', *American Health*, April 1994.)

'I'm completely low-risk for breast cancer,' I tell Anthony. 'This'll be some fatty tissue or something. The doctor's just going to tell me it's a virus and send me home again.'

'But it's growing,' Anthony insists one night, his unease tangible in the room. 'And it's so hard.'

'I know,' I answer this time. 'I'll make the appointment.'

I go to see our doctor on a Friday afternoon when my older children spend the weekend with their father. I take toys for two-year-old Elon and I pack my handbag with a supply of interestingly coloured drinks, ordinarily forbidden and absolutely guaranteed to distract him should the need arise. You see, he still breast-feeds. Stripping off my shirt in front of him and, worse, letting somebody else handle my breasts, is like inviting him to climb up and start suckling. At his age this is so rare a sight, it is more shocking than cancer in our society.

A lump, I tell the doctor. She can see it from several paces away, it's very apparent, and she feels it, tentatively. 'You need to be seen by a specialist. Within the next few days. Do you have private insurance? Make an appointment with whoever is available first.'

Here in the UK, where breast cancer is the second-biggest killer of women after lung cancer, although I can afford health insurance, I could choose not to pay for health care and rely on the State's universal provision of medicine. On the National Health Service, the doctor tells me, I would be seen within two weeks.

I have a notion that when something is serious it's safer to be in NHS hands – the Royal Free, a huge teaching hospital, is our local. 'No,' says my doctor, looking at me with her rather hard-edged expression, the stern one she uses on time-wasters, 'Your priority is to get diagnosed immediately.'

Somebody knocks on the doctor's office door, and she looks momentarily discomfited. 'It's Anthony,' my husband calls from outside.

'Oh, come in, come in,' our doctor calls. She turns to him with some enthusiasm. 'I've explained that Dina needs to see somebody straight away; I can't diagnose this,' she says. I think her manner's become subtly different, more relaxed, as if the men who consult her are more rational, more biddable than the women.

I have only ever been to doctors' appointments alone before, but this is just the first of several instances when I will listen, as if from a distance, as people talk over my head to my husband about my cancer.

Right now, though, I'm hardly looking at Anthony, barely noting the new long lines of worry that are already settling down into his face. Anthony has been profiled in *Vogue* magazine, where the writer Matt Seaton noted that 'his features are much more mobile in real life than comes across in photographs'. It's a good observation – you can read Anthony's feelings on his face, and over the coming months he will look increasingly drawn. But I'm angry, feeling my privacy encroached upon; we agreed he would set off for Cambridge to his eldest son Max's graduation, and I would report back on what the doctor said. Instead, here he is, in the doctor's office, and I'm furious.

Anthony's been ringing my mobile ever since I reached the surgery, and I haven't picked up, so he's made his own way over. Not that same afternoon, but some time later, while we still have the energy for these spats, we will have the first of many rows around this illness, and it goes something like this: 'You don't barge into my doctor's consultation' countered with, 'Your extreme desire for independence borders on the ludicrous.'

What happens this day is that we leave the office together, me urging him to set off for Cambridge – it is unspoken between us that I want him to get there before it is Shabbat, the Jewish Sabbath, twenty-five hours during which we don't drive, whereas his concern right now is my health. 'We can't do anything until Monday evening when I see the specialist. Go now, please, you don't want to miss Max's do,' I say.

Sara-Jenny, Marganit and Nina are at their father's house. So it's me, the baby and the breast with what now feels like a rectangular slab of metal embedded inside. When I first felt it, long ago in a bath one night, it was small and pea-shaped. This too-quiet afternoon at home is not after all a good time to have made the doctor's appointment. Our huge, airy house, that we were so lucky to find, with space for eight kids, their music and us, now feels like it's folding in on me.

I phone Elly. Apart from her five children, she has thirty-eight people coming for Friday-night dinner in two hours. Twenty minutes later she's at my door with two takeaway coffees and her own home-made cookies. (A tricky recipe, soft chocolate insides, dusted with icing sugar. My mother used to make these same chocolate crinkles, as they're called, and I often experiment, always trying to get them to taste right.)

Over the weekend, Elon feeds as usual. My appointment with the breast-cancer consultant is fixed for Monday evening. Elon doesn't drink much breast milk any more – maybe three minutes here, two minutes there – but it is whenever he wants.

And of course, last thing at night, before he goes to sleep.

'I'm tapering off,' I've told our scornful teenage brood, whose current mantra is, 'Do you know how embarrassing this is going to be for him when he's ten? Do you realize he's starting school soon?'

When I was pregnant with Elon, Chloë, my step-daughter, fourteen days older than Marganit, both girls aged eleven at the time, opened the topic at supper one evening. 'Dina,' she said. 'You're not going to do that thing, are you?'

'What thing?' I asked.

'You know, thingy in *Eastenders* tried it, that feeding of babies in public thing.'

'Not in public, Mum,' Marganit chimed in, very firm.

∞

It is 7.30 p.m. and I am Mr Al-Dubaisi's last patient on a day that began at eight o'clock with his NHS clinic, followed by meetings with other breast-cancer specialists and ending at this small hospital in northwest London.

Before touching my breasts, he studies them. He asks me to lift each arm separately over my head. Then he tells me to put my hands on my hips and press inwards, a procedure requested by each of the breast-cancer specialists I will see. Finally, he asks me to lie down and raise my arms again above my head, and this time he is not just looking, he feels the breasts for the first time, also prodding under my arms.

He turns away to let me get dressed, and the 'chaperone nurse' leaves the room, smiling goodbye. Back at his desk, Mr Al-Dubaisi says he's sending me for a mammogram, a scan and probably a biopsy. 'Yes, certainly, a biopsy,' he decides.

'What, tonight?' I say.

'Yes, yes, of course, tonight. Is your husband coming?' Anthony has stayed behind to settle Elon into bed, coming on to the hospital when our baby-sitter arrives.

I've had scans when pregnant, but I don't know what a mammogram or biopsy entails. I'm surprised it's all happening this same evening. A mammogram is an x-ray, Mr Al-Dubaisi explains, and a biopsy, he says, means putting a needle in. 'Very, very fine,' he says. 'I don't usually wait, but I will stay tonight to talk to you afterwards. For you,' he says. His voice is soft. It sounds to me like his way of letting me know it's serious.

I'm muddled. My older children won't be home from their father's until tomorrow. On Friday I told the children I was going to see our doctor – unusual enough for me – because, I guess, part of me knew this was a 'real' lump, while at the same time having only the sketchiest sense of breast cancer. When your children live in two homes, one of the things that needs attention is to make sure crucial stuff doesn't happen behind their backs. In the throes of divorce, I learned the key to guiding children through hard times is making sure you don't hide the bad things from them.

But this is all moving faster than I'd anticipated. The children not watching me leave home to go see a specialist, not being there when I get back from these tests – this is not what I planned. Like a crash course in breast-cancer diagnosis, this is all speeding now, relentlessly – wham, bam, mammogram.

Mr Al-Dubaisi tells me about the node. That's what he's been looking for under my arm, and he's found one: a bump he can feel, though I can't distinguish it even when he shows me where it is. It means the cancer is not confined strictly to the breast tissue, but shows signs of being on the move, seeping out of my breast, heading for the rest of my body. It's faster than me, then, because the concept of cancer spreading hasn't even entered my head yet, nor does it, really, even while Mr Al-Dubaisi says in the gentlest of voices, 'There is also a lymph node, Dina.'

Mr Al-Dubaisi wants three tests done, and this is happening right now, this evening, straight away. The bill for this first evening, paid for by my insurance, comes to £1547.50 – not including consultants' fees.

In the waiting area of the Garden Hospital, with its array of *Psychology Today* magazines and information about nicer noses, Anthony is sitting in an armchair, rigid, waiting; not, this time, knocking on the doctor's door to join the consultation. His anxiety is patent even before I head straight to him, distraught. 'I have to go right now for the tests . . . They're going to do a mammogram, that's an x-ray, a scan and a biopsy – what's a biopsy?' I say to Anthony. He shakes his head, almost unable to speak, when a nurse comes, tells me to get undressed, and put on a blue gown. 'Hang on,' I say, 'I don't understand exactly what's happening now.'

Her name is Jane, she is black and kind, her hair braided, little diamonds dotting her ears. 'You haven't had one of these before?' she asks.

'No,' I say, 'I haven't had anything.'

'Oh, well, first I do the mammogram, the x-ray. See, here is another lady just finished hers.' The woman looks closed, tense, and doesn't make eye contact.

The mammograph – a tall, thin, white metal machine with Plexiglas plates jutting forward from an upright beam – gets two kinds of press. The first hails it as a saviour, because it's able to detect cancerous cells in breasts two years before a doctor or self-examination would find anything. The other version says that mammography is big business; it's expensive, so it makes money for its producers, and that money would be better spent on researching the causes of cancer.

It's a machine designed by men, anyhow. You hoist your breast on to flat glass, no resting indentation curved for women, and then the upper plate is lowered on to the top of your breast to take the photograph. Jane eases the top plate down as slowly as her hand on the lever can do it.

'Why is the plate flat?' I ask, talking to cover my nervous anticipation of just what this steel plate is going to feel like when it hits its target and carries on pressing.

'They need the largest surface area possible, to get a good picture,' Jane tells me, sympathetically. It feels like being squeezed very tightly. A week from now, Jane will do this again, lowering the machine so slowly you can hear the air move, but by then my breast has had such a mauling, my second ever mammogram makes me faint.

The consultant radiologist, Dr Glenda Kaplan, is down the corridor in a tiny room, already bustling about as we come in. 'What do you do?' she asks, motherly, chatting.

'I interview children's authors for the *Guardian*,' I say.

'I mainly do breasts,' she replies. 'Since the screening programme (mammograms of women over fifty) started, it's ballooned.'

'No pun intended,' I say. She chuckles.

Like a bad lover, she spends about fifteen seconds on my left breast before heading for my tumorous right side where she lingers for a good twenty minutes, round and round with the scanner, bathed in its bluey gunge. 'I use warm gel,' she says, 'everybody seems to prefer it.'

'Ah, there it is,' she says, pointing out the cancer mass on the screen. It looks like all the baby scans I've ever seen.

'The black bit?' I hazard.

After the calm of the scan, watching hazy patches on a screen in a darkened room, the lights go on and Dr Kaplan and Jane flap a bit, getting ready. They weren't planning a biopsy this late on a Monday evening.

Anthony's at the end of the bed. 'It's all about distraction,' Dr Kaplan says to him. 'OK, you're going to have a local anaesthetic, first,' she tells me.

'Plenty of local anaesthetic,' I say.

'It makes a sound like a staple,' Dr Kaplan goes on, explaining the biopsy, a needle inserted into the tumour to suck out cancerous cells for diagnosis in a laboratory.

I'm looking away, hard. 'Keep very still, otherwise it will go in the wrong place.'

'I can feel it,' I say, not easy because I'm not moving anything, even my lips. Louder, I add, 'I can feel burning. Are you sure you've used enough anaesthetic? How do you know?'

I shut my eyes tightly, my fingers gripping Anthony's hand, my mind muttering grim, short sentences. It's all about distraction, this new reality. Narrow metal beds surrounded by breast specialists. Mr Al-Dubaisi says I need to stop feeding Elon. No way. No way is my August-born son going to be rushed into doing anything for which he's not ready – like being weaned.

One of the first things the older children said when we told them about the baby was, 'Due in August? Oh, poor thing – it'll be the youngest in the class.' August-born boys have a special place in the mythology: not only are they the youngest and likely to be the smallest in the playground, but also boys at that age are developing more slowly than the girls anyhow. There are whole books about how being born in August can affect your whole life.

I'm watching Dr Kaplan bandage my right breast after the biopsy. She lays a gossamer-thin piece of tape across the areas she's pierced, followed by a further layer of padding and then she seals my entire breast with a waterproof dressing that looks like clingfilm. Most of the breast is compressed now, including the nipple. It's Monday evening, and she's telling me not to have a bath until Thursday – to wash without getting the breast wet, and to make sure to keep the wound covered for three or four days, because of the risk of infection.

When things get tough, I run baths. I had two babies in the water, and it was the best way. So all I can think right now is, what, no bath? I notice her squashing my right nipple down beneath the bandage, but I don't register the consequences. I'm the breast-feeding expert in the room and I fail completely to see the problem ahead.

I do remember to say, half to Anthony, half to Dr Kaplan, 'So it's all right to feed Elon from the left side, then, is it?'

Which is when Dr Kaplan looks up sharply. 'You're breast-feeding, are you?'

'Ah, so that explains it,' she then says, half under her breath, but with a look on her face like a puzzle's been satisfactorily solved. 'The lactating pattern.' There were, she tells us, some grey zigzags on the ultrasound screen, manifestations of the milk-producing breast when its sound waves are reproduced as electronic images. Judging by the sound of Dr Kaplan's voice as she murmurs the words, reproduced visually as a trace of bemusement across her face, it seems she noted it mentally, while also dismissing it. It couldn't be, could it, given Elon's age?

'That's OK, isn't it?' I say now. 'I mean,' and something occurs to me for the first time, 'he can't catch cancer through the breast milk, can he?'

'No, no,' she answers, 'but you will have to stop, you know.'

I'm in pain from the biopsy she's conducted on my breast a few minutes before, so I just grimace and slide very gingerly off the bed. I'm used to people saying, 'You will have to stop, you know.' I have a houseful of older children daily insisting that Elon should quit being breast-fed.

'Yes, of course,' I say to Dr Kaplan, 'I'm tapering off.' She looks at me in some alarm, but I've seen that look before too.

I can breast-feed anywhere, and have done, including on top of a camel in the Sinai Desert. So what I'm thinking as I steady myself to head home this Monday night, is that it'll be fine, just feeding Elon from my left side, for the couple of nights or so till the bandage comes off the right. And, if he wants to feed from the right, now that I know it's medically safe, then that's no problem either. Yes, it may be tender, but I've breast-fed through the excruciating pain that is mastitis. So far, nothing I can't deal with here.

The older children are at their other parent, Elon is asleep and the baby-sitter is ensconced for a couple more hours. Anthony and I try to make this evening normal; we head out for a meal, stopping to buy some painkillers on the way.

It is just 10 p.m. when I walk through my front door. I've added some red wine and four Nurofens to the local anaesthetic Dr Kaplan administered.

As we cross the threshold, Elon has woken up, unusually for him. He's crying for 'meee', which is his language for breast milk. Through the stuffing in my mind I can hear his sad cries from downstairs, and the murmurs of Gabriella, our baby-sitter. I go upstairs and take him on my lap. I cuddle him and he moves instinctively to my right side. I say, 'Elon, can you see, Mummy has a bruise, I'm wearing a plaster, you can only drink from this other side tonight.'

'I will kiss it better, Mummy,' he says, easily shifting sides. Then, 'Did you trip over?' he asks. 'Sometimes I have a small bump,' he whimpers a few seconds later, before falling fast asleep.

By Wednesday morning I'm in real trouble.

Elon's crying on Monday night was the first sign of the temperature and illness that he develops over the next few days, which also means he is wanting to suckle much more than when in 'tapering-off' mode. My right breast, tightly bandaged, becomes more and more engorged, while he feeds almost steadily off the left side. Of course. Not only is he ill, not only does he know I have an impermeable bandage where only breast used to be, he can also tell there's some kind of intense interest being taken in his mother these days, and he's staking out his territory.

I phone Mr Al-Dubaisi to ask whether I can remove the dressing before three days are up. 'My breast is completely swollen, it's quite painful,' I tell him.

'Yes,' he says, 'yes, of course, just take it off.'

He is supposed to telephone me with the results from the biopsy on Thursday, but instead his secretary calls and says Mr Al-Dubaisi would like to see me and my husband later that day. She won't say why, just that 'he thought it would be nice if your husband came too'. I hang the phone back on its wall bracket and start crying for the first time. It's foreboding, and it's also about being shunted into a world where people address me in baby-talk: 'he thought it would be nice if your husband came too'.

It is Day Six. Yesterday Sara-Jenny turned sixteen. When she was born and I was out walking her to the park my head would be practically in the buggy with her, learning her face by heart. 'First baby?' a woman asked as she smiled at me in the street.

The first time I was due to leave her, I was completely unprepared for the feeling that hit me as I walked down the stairs from our flat. It was immensely powerful and struck without any warning whatsoever. One minute I was swinging down the path from my home, making my way to the station to catch a train, when it was as if an enormous band of elastic was gripping my shoulders, my waist, every vertebrae down my back, just pulling me home again. Nowhere on the *Guardian* Women's Page, compulsory reading throughout my adolescence, as far as I could remember, and nowhere in Penelope Leach's guide to motherhood, or not that I'd taken note of, did it say it was so hard to leave a baby.

But next week, Sara-Jenny and her three best friends are off to Europe – their first travels on their own, their first set of major exams, GCSEs, completed. A couple of weeks after that she will take off for a month, camping in Israel. She has finished her first eleven years of schooling, and never has to wear school uniform again. Today, though, she is home, with the others, for whom there are still some weeks of school, while Anthony and I go to see Mr Al-Dubaisi. Anthony's children, Chloë and Theo, are here too. Everybody is sprawled across the living-room rug and Elon is practising the break-dancing moves Sara-Jenny has taught him right in the way of older bodies trying to watch MTV. We leave with Theo peering steadily with one eye at the TV while Elon's bottom sits firmly over his remaining eye.

'You have a cancerous tumour,' Mr Al-Dubaisi tells me. He's watching my face closely. But this feels like news I already know. 'It's malignant,' he says emphatically. He's looking at me as if to say, do you understand?

'Some women come to me and say, remove it all, this is a diseased part of me, cast it off,' Mr Al-Dubaisi says, half to me, half to Anthony. As he talks, I have the feeling I am being monitored for my reaction, assessed to find out what manner of woman I may be.

'I'm quite attached to mine,' I say – a lame attempt at a pun, which completely passes by this doctor with his heavily accented English. All I mean is that it's integral to my body, not that easy to cast off.

'I know you are,' he says kindly.

In my case the lump is off-centre, apparently, so that may mean he can retain the nipple.

'And what about the long-term prognosis?' Anthony asks. 'Do you die from this?' It's the big question, quietly inserted.

'Nowadays,' the surgeon answers, steady, not rattled, 'even when we see seventy-five-year-olds, we think of them living for five or ten years. But because Dina is younger, I need to do better for her.'

Today has been the most fretful time. Ever since Mr Al-Dubaisi's secretary phoned at ten, to say the surgeon wanted to see me and my husband at five this afternoon I had been expecting the doctor to phone himself, and give me the results of the tests. I'm much more fixated on this slight than I am on the pros and cons of mastectomy, which is just a word to me, as is tumour for that matter.

In fact, I say to Mr Al-Dubaisi now, 'I wish you would have told me these results on the phone this morning. When we left Monday evening you said you'd have the results Thursday, and you'd call me with them.' The charade with the secretary, the being made to wait all day for a face-to-face appointment, feels aggravating. Or perhaps this is the first example of the famous anger. Once you have cancer, even strangers feel free to give you the advice that 'you need to expel your rage'.

'Professionally, I was not able to do that, Dina,' he says. 'I don't know your home circumstances, what situation you are in to hear this kind of thing,' he adds, turning to look at Anthony. Anthony's face is doing enough reacting for both of us; I feel a stab of pain as I see him reliving his father's death.

This is the difference. Anthony hears cancer, and thinks death. I have little experience of illness, and so all I'm thinking about is, OK, another blow to those hard-won routines, that chance to get some work done while the kids are at school. For me it's, right, I have to get through this, now when am I going to fit in all these appointments? Cut into my quiet time at home, and you cut into my sanity.

Mr Al-Dubaisi is already marking out my week. MRI scan tomorrow morning, and a bone survey on Monday. Monday is an all-day commitment, he's saying, because first they inject some radioactive fluid and then you have to wait three hours while it travels around the body, so your bones light up on the screen. It's called nuclear medicine.

'It is a very small amount of radiation, but of course you cannot breast-feed that day.' Finally, Mr Al-Dubaisi's voice penetrates my mind, which is spinning along the following lines: Elon needs picking up from nursery at twelve, Nina's school show is Monday afternoon . . . These are the last weeks of the summer term, least productive for the children but absolutely crammed with parental commitments to sports days, concerts and plays, so all day swanning around some hospital with green, glowing bones is out of the question.

I start to tell Mr Al-Dubaisi (he will call me by my first name, and I will call him Mr throughout) about the times I can and cannot do, and he stops me short.

'You need to understand that your health comes first for me, Dina. Right now it needs to come first. And you need to stop breast-feeding. The feeding is making the cells in the breast active.'

Now he is on my territory. I say, 'No, you don't understand, you can't just stop feeding a child, just like that. I am tapering it off. And I'm not feeding from the side which has the tumour.' I have said to Elon that Mummy's right side is not well, so he can just have the left breast. He wants to know when it will get better, but he is also quite content not to drink from it, even now the bandage from the biopsy is off.

'OK, OK,' the surgeon sighs. 'The other side, that's fine.' Seconds later it becomes obvious that it's not fine, after all. Mr Al-Dubaisi needs to do a physical examination. He wants to measure the tumour.

He looks startled when he sees the swollen state of my right breast. An engorged breast is like a rock full of tumours. It is huge, straining to contain the milk stored inside it, which has been sustaining a hefty toddler, and though it is stretched tight there are protrusions and bumpy areas.

'You're not expressing?' he asks, with concern.

'No,' I say, explaining as to a child. 'If I do that, then the milk production won't stop, and if you want me to stop feeding Elon, I have to let the milk dry up.' The end of breast-feeding is a painful process, however gradually you do it. As fast as the milk supply speeds up, it always seems to take longer to slow down, like it doesn't quite trust this capricious, momentary instinct of the baby to stop drinking, and it would rather keep full-on production for a few more days, just in case, than go to the trouble of cranking up the volume again should the baby change its still unformed mind.

'I see,' the consultant says. He tells me he can't feel the lump with his hands any more in this breast replete with milk. He's visibly disturbed by this; it is an interruption to his direct experience of the tumour. It means I will have to go back to Glenda Kaplan, so she can look at the lump on a scanner.

Back at his desk, he repeats that the breast-feeding will have to stop, that my health takes priority now. 'It is not that usual for two-year-olds to be breast-fed,' he says with a smile. 'It will not be a great deprivation for him.'

Sure, I think, but how do you stop? Every instinct in me says this is not the time to introduce sudden changes into Elon's life. And even if I do suddenly stop feeding him, what will I do when he's lying on the floor crying?

We leave Mr Al-Dubaisi's office and head down to x-ray where Dr Kaplan – luckily in the building – has been pre-warned by telephone and is ready and waiting to do the scan. Mr Al-Dubaisi wants to know the measurements of the tumour, information he'd prefer to glean through his hands, but, unable to get any sense of the lump because of my engorged breast, he is being forced to rely on the electrical method instead. Size, I'm slowly starting to understand, has some significance here. Two centimetres good, five centimetres bad, any bigger is a lot worse.

But Dr Kaplan has problems scaling this cancer, even with the latest scanner on the market. The oldest engineering in the world – the mechanism that says if the baby feeds solely from one breast then the other side will rise up in all its domineering might – defeats mere twenty-first-century technology. The cancer is flooded with milk, and no sound waves are penetrating. So Dr Kaplan gets back to basics herself. She digs her nails in where she thinks the borders of the tumour are, then checks on the screen to see whether her fingernail marks have shown up on the scan. Seven centimetres round, she makes it.

She runs her scanner across some of my organs at the same time. Something black shows up on the kidneys. 'I think it's probably nothing, but we'll check it out nevertheless.' Again, this is information the significance of which I don't really take in at that stage, just understanding that there will be some kind of further scan, using another type of machine, in yet another hospital.

Back upstairs Mr Al-Dubaisi says, 'The lymph node is mobile, this is good news. While it's still mobile, it's still very early days, the spreading is not established.'

'Do you mean the cancer hasn't spread?' Anthony asks.

'I can feel one mobile lymph node,' the surgeon answers. 'This is a sign of spreading, but now we need to do the further tests, the MRI, the bone scan, to see what has happened.'

I join the discussion at this point. 'It hasn't spread,' I say. Anthony looks at me, a lost look on his face. 'I know it hasn't spread,' I say again. 'I can tell.'

'That's good, instinct is good, your instincts are important,' Mr Al-Dubaisi says, looking up from where he is filling in boxes on various green sheets of paper ordering these different sets of diagnostic tests.

Then he says, again, 'Dina, you have to trust me, it is important that you trust me. The breast-feeding may be stimulating the cancer cells. Not many children his age are breast-fed; he will be OK.'

I look noncommittal, not even according him the civility he's just shown me by acknowledging my instincts on this matter are important. I grimace, albeit internally – what do doctors know?

That Thursday night – some hours after we come back from the hospital, after an evening talking with the children for the second time this week about the diagnosis and its implications, round our kitchen table dotted with boxes of Chinese takeaway food from Kaifeng, the kosher Chinese restaurant on our street – Nina has a nightmare. I am jerked out of sleep by her crying. 'You're not moving, are you, Mummy?' she says, when I come into the room she shares with Elon and sit next to her on the bed, stroking her arm. 'I dreamed we were all on a farm, everyone was there, Anthony, Max, Laura, everyone, and you said you just had to go off for a day, but you didn't come back.' She falls asleep as she finishes the sentence, and in the morning she doesn't even remember that she woke this night.

2. Tony Soprano, Eat Your Heart Out

After the diagnosis, the calm. We've had a week and a half of nonstop doctors' appointments, batteries of tests, and evenings with children wandering into the kitchen and saying, with marked pleasure, 'Ah, another takeaway', all culminating in the knowledge that size isn't everything, after all.

Seven and a half centimetres round, my tumour's a biggie, in cancer terms, the Tony Soprano of lumps. The kind the doctors thought wasn't just ruining the neighbourhood, but partying all over the city, spreading death and destruction.

Except that, remarkably – given its girth – this tumour hasn't spread to any of my organs. Glenda Kaplan's suspicions of the dark spot on my kidney turn out, within an hour and a transfer to a bigger hospital, to be baseless; it's scary-looking but harmless, just a patch of lumpy stuff packing no fire power.

The cancer is contained in my right breast and, so far as can be detected before cutting me open, one lymph node. And my lymph node is mobile, still dodging around, throwing punches, fighting back. More good news. Stationary lymph nodes are the ones with their feet in cement blocks.

This process of finding out how far the cancer has travelled is called 'staging' by the doctors, who tend to use these phrases with a sideways glance across the desk. If I don't remember to ask, my brain only processing the language a couple of hours after words are spoken, then the medical people – not great at explaining procedures – seem to leave you to find out what's happening as you go along. I ask Mr Al-Dubaisi what 'staging' is, but neglect to find out just how an MRI is conducted.

As I lie on my back for the MRI, I think how lucky it is I watch *ER* on TV, or I wouldn't even know I'm about to be slid backwards into a tunnel. Thanks to television, I also know I'm at risk of feeling claustrophobic, only I don't. The main sensation inside the tunnel is of light, a white light with a blue line running down the middle of it.

So far, so smooth. But then I am rolled forward again into ordinary hospital light, for another bit they haven't explained. 'Small jab,' a guy called Matt is saying to me from somewhere near my toes, as he approaches the scanning bed. He has to inject some fluid into my veins to make my organs show up on the screen. 'I'll just put this right in,' Matt says, but seconds later he is still bashing away ineffectually at my veins, the ones in his own forehead throbbing with the repressed anxiety of it all. 'I'll call Dr Kaplan,' he tells me, 'if I don't get it in this time.' And then, 'I won't turn you into a pincushion, I promise.'

He leaves the room for a while, then comes back in and says, 'I haven't forgotten you.'

'No,' I answer, mean, lips tight, 'I haven't forgotten you either.'

'You're doing really well,' he says, before scurrying out of the room again.

Many, many months later I will be invited to a meeting at the Houses of Parliament, with a man they call the Cancer Tsar. Mike Richards is in charge of designing five-year cancer plans for government spending. One of the topics that keeps coming up during the course of this round-table discussion between drugs-company representatives, medical professionals, cancer charities and me is the question of whether money is wisely spent on 'teaching communications skills to doctors'.

'We allocated one million pounds to communications training,' one of the participants says.

I listen, open-mouthed. 'You're joking,' I say at the meeting, with all the eloquence at my disposal. 'Doctors are just rubbish at communicating.' People round the table grin, a little uncomfortably.

'I think that being a doctor requires such a high level of detachment,' I explain. 'You know, being a surgeon, cutting into people's flesh, or even just giving repeated injections. But communicating takes empathy, the opposite of detachment. I'm just not sure it's possible for that much detachment to coexist with the kind of mind that communicates well. So it cannot be sensible to spend money on a pointless cause.' The long, rectangular table of politicians and medical professionals smile into their note pads and move on to another topic.

When Matt finally gives up and sends for Glenda Kaplan, she limps into the room nursing a bruised knee and inserts the needle painlessly and in one swift move. She tells me she has been canvassing second opinions from her hospital colleagues this morning about her leg. 'One tells me it's a strain, the other one's saying it's something else and needs investigating,' she tells me, shrugging. That's second opinions for you, we both laugh. Later, when I'm changing back into my clothes after the scan, she comes into the cubicle to say the MRI is clear – no cancer has spread into the organs. 'Normally we don't give this news straight away,' she says. 'But . . .' It is a kindness.

We go to Wimpole Street in London's West End for the bone scan, which I am assured will finish in time for me to catch Nina's school show back in Hendon, while Elon is picked up from nursery by Anthony's mother. I'm feeling nauseous these days because Mr Al-Dubaisi has prescribed what seem like enormous tablets for me to swallow whose remit is to dry up my supply of breast milk, but it's a sunny day and Anthony and I are having yet another long drive on our own. The up-side of the raised tension and its consequent squabbling is that these drives to different hospitals and hours spent in waiting rooms just talking feels almost like holiday time, time out.

This time I know there's a needle ahead. Mr Al-Dubaisi has explained I will be injected with radioactive fluid, whatever that means.

'You off to Australia?' the guy at reception says, bronzed himself from a trip to Brazil, and thinking we're next in the queue for immunization. 'No,' Anthony says grimly, 'bone scan.'

Walking into a room bearing the doorplate NUCLEAR
MEDICINE, you do wonder what's on the other side:
Hiroshima? In fact it's a woman doctor who came here
from Iran thirty-four years ago. She can see I'm anxious
about the needle, but she just smiles at me and says, 'I
have lots of experience,' and in fact while I'm busy bracing myself for her not getting the vein first time, and
having to do the procedure all over again, she has already
inserted the needle. (Twenty-one months later I come
back to this same room for the same procedure, but by
then my veins are so battered from repeated injections
she takes one look and calls in a superior.)

'You are now radioactive,' she tells me. 'So you must
stay away from pregnant mothers and small children for
twenty-four hours.' I make a face. This reminds me of
when doctors prescribe ointment for children's eye infections, which you are somehow supposed to insert into the
lower lid of your small child's eyes. The instructions say,
'insert three times a day', but they never tell you how
exactly you're supposed to get a small, squirming eyelid to
relax long enough to squirt ointment inside.

Staying away from my boisterous, cuddling small boy
is equally implausible – I'm not supposed to have him on
my lap. Really? Elon has already said this morning, 'I
don't want you to have any more doctors' appointments,
Mummy.'

But that is later. For now, there are three hours to
spend in the West End, Marylebone High Street specifi-
cally, probably London's best shopping road.

I return to the nuclear-medicine room swinging shopping bags. Back on a narrow table, arms strapped to my

side as I slide under a monitor, I get to see my skeleton on a screen, no black spots, while the doctor chats away about her building problems and questions Anthony closely about the pros and cons of suing the building profession. I am radioactive but bone-healthy, and back in Hendon in time for Nina's show.

'Staging' done and dusted, I'm thinking a day out. Really, I want a day in, I want my life back, with its quiet mornings when the house is empty. They say it's an intrusive disease, but they don't explain that part of the intrusion is because of the nonstop medical appointments, the incessant disruption of my hard-won routines of children at school, men at work, and quiet mornings in which to write.

Failing the return of my pre-cancer life, however, some grade-A distraction will also do. Anthony and I are invited to a headline-making, paparazzi-heavy function this coming Tuesday morning. I am trying out my fifteenth outfit. It's the opening of the Diana Memorial Fountain, and Anthony – Princess Diana's lawyer – is supposed to be there. Having taken two weeks off work himself to shepherd me back and forth to doctors' appointments, he would actually like an ordinary day's toil safe behind his desk, but I'm insisting on attending the Diana event, and I'm the one with cancer.

Then Mr Al-Dubaisi calls us in for a consultation. Now he knows the extent of what he's dealing with it's time to start the first stage of my treatment: chemotherapy. I am having chemotherapy before surgery in an attempt to reduce the size of the lump in my breast. Mr Al-Dubaisi has arranged for me to meet the oncologist in charge. The appointment is for Tuesday morning, the same as the Memorial opening.

'Can't do Tuesday morning,' I say.

Anthony butts in, 'Tuesday's fine.'

'No, really,' I smile winningly. 'Any other time, except Thursday that is, another school show, but any other time at all.'

'Dina,' my surgeon says, 'I have explained many times, it is important now that your health comes first. For me, that is the prime concern. We must start treatment as soon as possible, so you must attend these appointments. There is a series of events we must set in motion.'

'Of course,' Anthony tells him, 'Tuesday morning is fine.'

'OK,' I say, 'but I want you to know Anthony's standing up the Queen for this.'

Pause. Mr Al-Dubaisi looks up. 'Really?'

'Yes, really,' I say. The surgeon looks at Anthony, his deeply entrenched medical self-assurance now compromised by a semi-comical, semi-quizzical mix of, 'is this what passes for Dina-style wit?' Anthony confirms the royal connection and, what do you know, suddenly my health is so D-list, it wouldn't get a table at a roadside café, let alone the Ritz.

'Well,' Mr Al-Dubaisi says grinning, 'I don't want to be a spoilsport.'

We've only known him for a week or so but Mr Al-Dubaisi often makes us smile. His heavily accented wryness, stuff like, 'Your intuition is very useful Dina, but – for my own peace of mind – we will undertake the diagnostic examinations nevertheless,' delivered deadpan.

This, though, this complete volte-face, from a man who's been trampling roughshod over every priority in my life on the grounds that for now and the foreseeable future my health is the only consideration, this sudden indication that an elderly lady in matching coat and shoes knocks my health for six in the Al-Dubaisi universe, this makes Anthony and me laugh out loud. As fast as Mr Al-Dubaisi has given us the new permission to skip appointments, so we both lose any desire at all to place anything before my proceeding with the steps towards treating this disease.

The several subtle, but eye-catching and breast-requiring, little numbers go back in the cupboard. Anthony does his five-minute interview for the BBC's *Today* programme about the fountain (which he has never seen, has had no involvement with, and for which he bears no responsibility) from our home, with Elon calling out in the background, instead of being recorded from Hyde Park, with the sound of the fountain as backdrop. And come 10 a.m. Tuesday morning I'm wearing the same old easy-to-pull-off top – my newly *de rigueur* outfit for medical examinations – to meet Peter Ostler, consultant oncologist.

He looks extremely young – though it turns out he's around the same age as me, late thirties, early forties, as in fact, is Mr Al-Dubaisi. We would all three have graduated around the same time, but now I'm in a risk category that counts my survival in five-year steps.

While Mr Al-Dubaisi radiates seniority, Peter Ostler springs into the room, long and gangly like a teenage boy. Mr Al-Dubaisi wears thick, tailored suits that speak expense and gravitas; Peter Ostler wears natty checked shirts and blue jackets over dark trousers, and lopes through the hospital corridors like he's crossing the veldt. We meet at Mount Vernon, a large hospital with a specialist cancer unit. It's in a part of the world I rarely get to, and the first few times we get lost travelling there. At the bottom of my road, you can either turn left and go deeper into suburbia, or you can branch off and join a motorway, the M1. The fastest way for me to reach Mount Vernon is to travel five junctions'-worth of the M1, leaving the highway for an outer suburb of leafy, wide roads, some closed off with private gates. It feels like going to the countryside, and I pride myself on being a city girl, by nature anyhow.

The hospital itself is a collection of buildings, some edged in fake timber, linked by signs denoting their intellectual or financial genesis, names like 'Marie Curie research centre', or 'Paul Strickland scanner unit'. Parts of it are very old, with the feel of a Victorian asylum, tiled corridors and green paint, other bits brand new, all carpet tiles and cream paint. Down bleak corridors, sitting out on long, boring lawns, in the cafeterias, there are clones: people without hair. Egg-shaped heads minus distinguishing features; well, all except the fact that some are smoking. Size (even of tumours) may not be a definitive marker, I hear myself thinking bleakly, but hair sure does count.

Peter Ostler is conducting a trial of cancer treatments – much is still experimental. He asks me if I'll participate, and I leap at it, saying, 'Yes, great' as soon as he raises the subject.

'Uh, hang on,' he says, looking a little alarmed, 'there's

a procedure. You need to have it explained first, need to know the research protocols.'

On trial are two different chemotherapy recipes: Adriamycin plus Cyclophosphamide (AC for short), and Taxotere (T). So, the trial's name is TAC, and the idea of it is to find out whether it makes a difference in which order the drugs are given. But precedence isn't all that is at stake here; in 2004, when I first begin chemotherapy, Taxotere is not yet universally used in the UK, although Taxotere-based chemotherapy is preferred by US doctors. The AC combination works out at around £800 a shot, while Taxotere costs over £2000 every time it's injected. Money, it turns out, also matters.

Taxotere, trials have found, lowers the chance of breast cancer returning to women whose nodes are affected: a 27.5 per cent reduction, to be precise. This disease feels like it is cutting a swathe through Western women – leaving us single-breasted, no-breasted, falsely breasted – but when doctors talk about new drugs there is a sense that we breast cancer sufferers are also, increasingly, alive.

So, doctors, convinced of the effectiveness of Taxotere, now want to refine their use of the potent ingredient. They're working out how many doses, in combination with which other drugs, and at what point in the treatment schedule, the use of Taxotere can be optimized.

I know all this because when Dr Ostler asks if I'll join an experiment, I say yes, immediately, and then Anthony starts asking questions. I heard trial, and thought, good, anything that turns this into something more than being ill. Anthony is very anxious – what if the trial compromises my treatment? Unlike NHS patients, for whom

Taxotere is not yet approved (though it's been passed in the States since 1998), as a private patient my doctors can prescribe chemotherapy gold dust if they choose. So Anthony wants to know what is the point of my joining a trial, which may carry risks; obviously if you're trying out two different regimes, half the people on the experiment are getting the prescription that's going to be least effective?

Dr Ostler is keen to recruit me to the trial – in another conversation he says, with some irritation, that all patients should be in trials, so answers would be found faster – but he adds that if, at any stage, the team of himself, Mr Al-Dubaisi and Glenda Kaplan decide I need a different kind of treatment, they'll remove me from the regime. (But Anthony is right: months later, the doctors give me a choice, and the decision I make is partly influenced by not wanting to 'spoil' the TAC study.)

At home, I'm trialling alternatives to breast milk. My top concern these days is easily summed up: how do you stop, how do you stop? One friend says, 'I think you just say, Mummy can't feed you any more, and you offer other things – a cuddle, a sweet treat.'

I remember a (male) doctor telling me that 'once they see steak and chips, they just lose interest in breast-feeding'. Not true, actually, but chocolate milk in a bottle does work and remarkably – to me, anyhow – pretty soon Elon is taking the change of menu in his stride. A little resigned, sure, and even a little fed up, but basically good-natured about it. 'Mummy can't feed you any more,' I say, keeping my shirt firmly tucked, and his hands clasped in mine, stopped mid-exploration.

His face says, 'Huh, adults.' Then, a good kid, he makes a joke out of it, giggling as he says, 'Well, can I still squash it, Mummy, your breast? Or can I bite your cheek instead?' He laughs out loud at that one. And so do I. Good joke. 'Can I bite your nose?'

I'm still chuckling about this, now, forty-eight hours after meeting Dr Ostler, a day after phoning him to say, 'I have thought it over, I'm in.' Then I stop laughing, fast. I am lying rigid because I forgot to ask the one question that might have made me think twice about becoming a medical guinea pig, a nicety of the procedure that I didn't cross-question the doctor about, and now it's happening.

It's cold, and I'm wearing one of these blue hospital wraps that gape open at the back, so I'm already shivering before I go in to the tiny day operating room. 'I'll be doing the biopsies under local,' Dr Kaplan says.

'What do you mean, biopsies?' Too late, I'm sharp, on the ball with the questions. 'I thought it was one biopsy. Do you mean you're doing more than one?'

To join the trial the biopsy I've already had is not enough. Trial HQ, over in the States, needs more bits of my tumour. Peter Ostler has told me this, but definitely uses the word 'biopsy', singular.

Here I am, once again, flat on Dr Kaplan's couch. I've dropped Elon at nursery, rushing because my appointment with Dr Kaplan is for nine-thirty so I'll have time to do the biopsy, recover and get back to nursery in time to pick Elon up at twelve-thirty. My sense of this cancer is still that I slot it into available gaps, not that it is going to require its own allotted time.

Once in the room, lying on the narrow, white-sheeted

bed, with the long strip of blue paper towel that comes freshly off a roll for each new patient, Dr Kaplan chats away softly, filling cold silences. These rooms are always chilly, she says, busying herself, setting up her equipment, adjusting her chair. And then she says, 'I'll be doing the biopsies under local.'

'How many biopsies?' I'm on my back, in a gown that gapes open, and I'm trying to sound assertive.

'Three,' she says.

Dr Ostler's research nurse is in the room too. 'Do you understand about the trial?' she asks me, in a voice that reaches my now hyper-anxious ears as extraordinarily patronizing.

'Yes,' I say.

'Has it been explained to you?'

'Yes.' I'm abrupt, barking out my replies, and struggling to sit up.

'Sorry, you're disadvantaged lying there,' she says.

Dr Kaplan takes over, her gentle stream of information more frenetic as she sees the pain on my face. 'I can't put local anaesthetic right into the tumour,' she tells me.

'I don't want to know that, I don't want to know that,' I say.

Under her breath she mutters, 'Why ever couldn't they use the original sample?'

One lone school of cancer thought opposes screening programmes because the still relative inefficiency of mammograms means that for every tumour discovered, hundreds of women endure false scares and biopsies. To me, a biopsy is so painful my late-night conversation with friends these days is to ask what kind of person they think it takes to plunge a needle into an unanaesthetized part of a woman's breast.

After Dr Kaplan has finished, the samples sealed in a test tube and placed in a small, insulated freezer box to be sent to America, I sign the trial papers giving my consent to joining the trial, and claiming that I understand what's involved. I then walk down the corridor to have a further mammogram and crumple to the floor.

One minute I'm perched on the chair, waiting for the nurse to come back into the room, the next I have fallen forward, sliding down to the tiled floor in the small room containing the mammograph. The nurse comes back in, sees me, helps me to sit upright, and then goes off to bring me some tea, along with the information that Dr Kaplan is on her way. But I stand up, walk out into the reception area, where the magazine I was reading before the biopsy is still lying open on the same page, climb the one flight of stairs, and leave the hospital. It feels like the first bit of control I take over this illness, an iota of defiance against these passages of initiation into the Amazons. I'm muttering the word as I drive away, mazon means breast in Greek, doesn't it, and the 'a' is not-breasted; they cut off their right breasts so they could shoot arrows better . . . the words are shafts in my head. I'm just beginning to realize that I don't want to be this brave.

3. The Cancer Victim Who is Out and About

This is odd. I look fine. I've had a haircut, one of the snippets of advice I've actually absorbed from the chemotherapy information leaflet somebody, somewhere, handed me during the past few weeks. Shorter hair hangs in there longer apparently, survives the drug onslaught better. Sarah, who has been through this with her mother, cuts my hair. I go to her flat instead of the salon, because I suppose I don't feel like having the breast-cancer chat in a room pulsing with other people's healthy lives.

Sarah's been cutting Meg Rosoff's hair too – a children's author Penguin Books publicity team has been promoting for months. The last few times I've seen Sarah she's told me how one of her other clients has been given the most fantastic book deal for a children's novel, but I didn't make the connection between the hair chatter and the barrage of press releases about Rosoff that have, for weeks now, landed on my desk in drifts as thick as the hair coming off my head right now. Finally, it all comes together. 'Oh, Meg Rosoff! Sure, she's written this book, *The Way We Live Now*.'

This is the way we live now. Rosoff is nearing the end of

her chemotherapy, as I am starting mine. In Sarah's 60s-style living room on top of a West End pub, there is concentration and concern underlaid with anxiety on her face, as we both look at my hair in the mirror. Sarah's mother has just passed the five-year mark since being diagnosed, and she is treating what's starting to look like a line of clients. As we talk, her scissor steel flashing, it feels like she is at the point of an infinite trail of women, using an ancient skill to try to ward away the evil illness. She cuts with flair, making new angles appear on my face, so I skip down the stairs from her flat – this illness can't catch me-eee.

Back in Hendon, I cycle everywhere, with Elon strapped into a child seat on the back of my bicycle, like a miniature Chinese emperor surveying the masses. I believe you can negotiate physical ordeals, such as the chemotherapy starting next week, by getting fit. It's how I dealt with pregnancy and childbirth – keep moving, beat the fatigue.

So I look great: fresh skin and short, swingy haircut. People in my neighbourhood have started to hear about the cancer. And this is the strange bit. Am I supposed to be ill in bed? People look startled when they see me. I feel like 'the cancer victim who is out and about'. Whispering acquaintances ask Anthony how I am.

But there is one living room where there are no sideways glances, no sotto voce mutters, where everything life throws out is dealt with directly and openly. No secrets here, and no taboos either. My friend Elly takes me round to Hendon's best 'shaitel lady', the local woman who sells wigs from her home.

In my Orthodox Jewish community many of the married women cover their hair for religious reasons. In fact, I'm the only one of my parents' four daughters whose hair shows. As it happens, the first time I married, I did keep my straight, chestnut-brown hair covered, for a while, sometimes with a wig, mostly with berets and scarves.

Back then, I worked on the features desk of the just-founded newspaper, the *Independent*, and my boss had lost her hair to alopecia. So, for quite different reasons, we two had a range of methods for covering our heads. One day we both came in wearing berets, and Marie Helvin, who was writing a style piece for us, turned up sporting a beret too. I remember Andreas Whittam Smith, the *Independent*'s editor, strolling over – as section heads often did when Helvin appeared. 'Ah,' Whittam Smith said amiably, 'this must be the new fashion then, berets.' Shortly after that I chucked all head-coverings into the bin.

My parents, who live in Israel, don't know I have this cancer – we speak rarely. These days, though, the doctors keep asking me for family medical details, incidences of cancer, details I just don't have, although when I give my now-standard reply, 'I'm not really in contact with my family,' the doctors immediately tell me it's fine, not to worry. I register with a kind of bemusement that there's a part of me that thinks if I phone my mother and father and give them the news that I am this ill, then they will deal with it for me. That my parents will 'make it all better', in that legendary way parents are supposed to.

This illness, with its cure that attacks hair, has connotations for me way beyond the medical. There is also the fact that Ashkenazi Jewish women, like myself, can carry two genes that – when mutated – cause breast cancer: BRCA1 and BRCA2. It is bizarre to me that these genes are named as they are, because the abbreviation sounds like *bracha* – Hebrew for blessing. I think of them as *bracha* one and *bracha* two, and any day now I'm going to find out where the blessing lies.

It's pouring with rain the night I go for my wig-fitting. A young woman opens the door. To the right is a room filled with hairpieces, bright lights, a big mirror and a large swivel chair. Though both cover their hair, neither of the women in charge wears a wig; one is in a snood, the other a kerchief.

The wigs on display are not ready-styled. There are bins full of hanks of (mainly dark) human hair, which has been hand-sewn on to netting – laborious work, done by women in other countries, before the wigs are sent to the West. Human-hair wigs, as different from the synthetic kind as a Harold Pinter play from reality TV, are expensive, costing well over a thousand pounds. But for that you get a wig with a parting that can be brushed through and moved, that doesn't lie rigidly in one artificial line, and is cut to your shape. A friend, in hospital with leukaemia, wears one of these wigs, and the nurses remark on its realism.

The women here are very kind in a businesslike way. They spend a long time matching hair colour, giving advice, getting it right. During the evening many other women come in, wigs looking so wrong on their heads they look almost like men in drag, until the *shaitel* lady tweaks, cuts, styles and they leave, their chic renewed.

A soon-to-be bride is fretting, and hours, literally, are spent, offsetting finite shades of almost-black against her snow-white complexion. Either too dark or too light, and the wig hair, no matter that it is human and not artificial, immediately looks obviously fake. Though the girl's mother and aunt are both involved in the discussion, as are other friends who pass through, there is an air of sadness here, a passing on of a burden, this wig-wearing.

The ultimate wig colour is located for me too, minute comparisons of grades of chestnut colouring made. These women are patient as time. But no surprise either, that back in Elly's car, the weight of this evening suddenly overwhelms, and with the rain still beating down on the windscreen, I sit dissolved in tears, Elly silent and sympathetic, her own bewigged head in her hands.

I carry make-up with me at all times now, so in our driveway I camouflage the red eyes and walk back into our house, brandishing the wig. Nina looks shell-shocked when she sees it, while on the older girls' faces I think I discern a mix of emotions, including an undercurrent of welcoming the wig because at last their mother will 'fit in' around Hendon.

Anxious about how this physical manifestation of the illness will affect the children – this likelihood that I will become bald – I am deliberately forward about showing the wig to the children straight away; 'dealing' with it, making it a wide-open issue. Within seconds all this parental management proves to be completely beside the point, because a hurtling mass of energy hurls himself on me, grabs the shiny, gleaming and just-expertly-cut hank of hair from my hand and, roaring with belly-laughs, prances round the house wearing my new hair. Elon has – in a life I have largely dedicated to entertaining and stimulating him with the best of experiences, the richest of toys – never seen anything which makes him laugh quite so raucously as this brand new plaything Mummy's brought home tonight.

For me, friends have started bringing books about breast cancer. Well-meaning stuff about the mind-body connection, and tracts of nutritional advice. The books start coming almost as soon as the food. It is the second way people respond – those who are able to respond – when they hear you have cancer. I think they bring food because they want to nourish you.

The books are different; the books are about empowerment. People have fixed ideas about cancer, the main one being that cancer is not just a physical illness, not just about cells dividing too rapidly – though this is a proven, known fact, as incontestable as the earth's roundness – but that it is somehow a psychologically rooted disease, that the mind has some role to play in fighting cancer.

Above all else, people seem to believe you will have a better chance of surviving cancer – that disease of the body to which as yet no complete cure has been found – if you can 'take control' of your illness. Information-gathering is supposed to be one of the prime ways of doing this; like squirrels bustling about to collect nuts to ward off winter's harshness, so hoarding and wielding knowledge about your options is supposed to strengthen you against cancer's ravages, is actually supposed to lessen the chances of the cancer returning.

I don't believe this myself. But I prove as vulnerable to people's gifts as I am to breast cancer, and so I read the books left on my doorstep, or offered in packages with cakes and flowers. The ones about how your personality predestines you for cancer. Like overdosing on too many women's magazines personality quizzes at once, I now know I am too angry, too controlling, too repressed, and my upbringing wasn't up to much either – but also that I find it difficult to say no, I am incurably unassertive. So naturally I also read the numerous texts about what foods poison you and which ones heal, and, my own personal favourite, *Breast Cancer for Dummies*, one of a series of books more usually aimed at computer users.

It is the books that first make me feel fear – a pointless emotion in these circumstances. Immune to doctors' grave looks, I turn out to be porous to print.

One book changes that and gives me back my balance. Anthony lays an offering on my desk called *Bathsheba's Breast: Women, Cancer and History*, by James S. Olson (The Johns Hopkins University Press).

Olson is a professor, chair of the history department at Sam Houston State University. He wrote the book as a response to losing his left hand and forearm to cancer – having first chosen to try simply removing the tumour, followed by radiotherapy, as opposed to amputation, before the return of the tumour (twice) forced him towards the final loss. 'The choices,' he writes, 'seemed so bewildering, so vague and imprecise. Scientists, I naively thought, ought to be different from historians, less likely to debate an issue and traffic in contrasting personal opinions.'

But when writing about the subject, Olson made, as he says, a historian's choice, opting to explore breast cancer rather than the soft-tissue sarcoma that attacked him, because, he writes, 'throughout much of human history breast cancer was cancer, and prominent women who endured the disease left behind a rich paper trail'. Well before treatment begins, I am already talking to the *Guardian* newspaper about shredding my own paper trail, documenting this illness in a fortnightly column, so this sentence feels like it's addressed directly to me.

But it's Olson's next sentence that clinches it for me and makes this my manual: 'The gender dynamics of the disease – female patients and male physicians – have also been a constant over time, shaping perceptions of the disease and its treatment.' The barrier between me and this book was its male author; with his pinpointing of this issue, like all the others he analyses – the quacks, the talk about a cancer personality, the doctors' (continued) stumbling in the dark – he punctures my reserve. For me, gender courses through my sense of my breast-cancer story: my breast-feeding son, my male doctors and their tendency to look over to Anthony to confirm some thought or other, other women's response to this illness. So when Olson talks of the gender dynamics of the disease, it feels like I'm chatting to somebody who speaks my inner language. So far, as a patient, that sensation has been remarkably rare. Most often, I am struggling to decipher what the doctors are saying and, moreover, what they are not saying.

I read *Bathsheba's Breast* almost in one sitting, and then find myself returning to it often, looking stuff up. I realize one of the things I find so comforting about it is that it offers genuinely informative background, and that is all. The relief is huge. Here is one book that is not about making decisions, there is no guilt riding on whether I can stand soya milk for the rest of my life, or whether if I drink my ordinary coffee without really looking at it, then it doesn't count towards hastening my death from this illness. *Bathsheba's Breast* is simply context, like hearing a particularly intelligent parliamentary debate without any vote riding on it. Nice, you know; a distraction from the shrill and conflicting cancerama babble currently sited in piles around the rest of my desk.

Also, the history of breast cancer, à la Olson, is gripping. Breast cancer is the one you can see, of the more than 200 differing versions of this disease, the lump that's on the surface. Egyptian medics 3500 years ago described bulging tumours in the breast. The mastectomy is equally ancient; in 548 AD Aetios of Amida, physician to the Byzantine court wrote: 'I make the patient lie down and then I incise the healthy part of the breast beyond the cancerous areas and I cauterize the incised parts. Then I again incise and excise the breadth from its depths and I again cauterize the incised area. And I repeat the procedure often.' Mr Al-Dubaisi uses the word 'excise' all the time, the only person of my acquaintance to do so, and I have to ask him what it means the first time he says it. To be reminded that anaesthesia did not come until the 1840s, though, is the most painful of history lessons.

Olson traces a timeline from the oldest cases of breast cancer to the current day, taking in all the celebrity names along the way, from the lovers of emperors to Nancy Reagan. He records the roots of the ideas that it came from 'black bile' and the mad nutritional theories, as well as the chauvinism of the personality prognoses.

This is enlightening stuff, light which is refracted on to other areas of female medicine: like the surgeons who insisted that it was morally beneficial for women to feel pain during surgery (and did somebody mention the word childbirth?). As late as 1850 Benjamin Hill, a Boston surgeon, Olson records, tried to get breast cancer patients to accept cauterizations of their tumours without anaesthetics. Hill lauded the virtues of 'pain as moral medication'. Not until the 1890s were surgeons willingly using anaesthesia on every patient.

The backbone of the text charts the history of the arguments over mastectomy and then radical mastectomy, and the muddle of scientific opinion. 'In fact,' Olsen says, 'eighteenth-century physicians knew only a little more about the causes of breast cancer than Hippocrates and Galen and only a little less than contemporary oncologists.'

Because he is, first of all, a historian, he *describes*; so he doesn't say what I am newly, and shockingly, discovering to be the case: that there's more profit in finding a cure than in working out the cause. Drugs companies rise and fall on the stock market according to their shares in the latest 'magic bullet' advance – but work out what's causing the rise in cancer in our times, and maybe we won't need those medicines. It doesn't feel like a cause that should be too hard to elucidate: take Japanese women with their low rates of cancer, and move them to

Ohio – within two generations their cancer incidence has risen. Mr Al-Dubaisi talks often about the Japanese, and how little, he says, they suffer from even lung cancer, though Japanese men are notoriously heavy smokers. Breast cancer has doubled since the 1970s; every three minutes in the United States a woman is being diagnosed.

What Olson's book reveals is how the treatments – surgery, chemotherapy and radiotherapy – have been the subject of debate and swerving opinions for as long as they have existed. How each famous woman of recent times who has made the personal decision about which course to pursue has had to endure media scrutiny followed by criticism over how her choice influences others in the same situation. My generation may be the last, or perhaps the one before the last, to die of this disease.

Olson writes about the *Oxford English Dictionary*'s definition of cancer, unchanged since 1889. It reads: 'A malignant growth or tumour in different parts of the body that tends to spread indefinitely and to reproduce itself and also to return after removal; it eats away or corrodes the part in which it is situated and generally ends in death.' As the century changed, and more and more drugs to control cancer have become available, the editors of the *OED* were contacted by Macmillan Cancer Research, who urged a rewriting of the hundred-year-old entry. The campaigners wanted something on the lines of: 'What happens when a group of cells grows in a disorderly way and invades neighbouring tissues. They may or may not later spread into distant parts of the body.'

On Wikipedia, the online encyclopedia edited by all,

this shift away from language like 'corrosive' and 'eats away' has been taken up. Wikipedia says: 'If untreated, cancers may eventually cause illness and death, though this is not always the case,' and, 'Once referred to as "the C-word", cancer has a reputation for being a deadly disease. While this certainly applies to certain particular types, the truths behind the historical connotations of cancer are increasingly being overturned by advances in medical care. Some types of cancer have a prognosis that is substantially better than nonmalignant diseases such as heart failure and cerebrovascular accident/stroke.'

The entry in the online and multiple-volume edition of the *OED* has yet to be changed – established dictionary processes grinding more slowly than medical ones. One non-hospital morning, I sit at my desk, a gesture in the direction of my previous life, and make some journalistic phone calls, chasing the trail of this process of defining cancer. So John Simpson, editor-in-chief of the *OED*, tells me, 'It's all to do with cycles of revision; there are many definitions that long ago needed updating. At the moment we're working on P.'

4. The Raspberry-Coloured Fluid

*n*obody mentions amnesia as a side effect. But in the middle of the night I remember that it's Anne Fine I'm interviewing. Perplexing emails have been coming from colleagues at the *Guardian* about whether I should be doing an interview this week, to which I reply that I'm not. Suddenly, I wake, bolt upright, the whiteboard in my head blank no longer: oh, yes, I am due to meet and question an ex-children's laureate. To top that, for days I've been thinking Anthony's birthday is a week away at least, only (yikes!) today is Wednesday, and his birthday is this Friday.

Today is my first chemotherapy. First of the 'third Wednesdays', latest of the black dates to enter my mental calendar. Second Thursdays my girls go to their father, now third Wednesdays are for cancer treatment.

Though it feels like a previous existence, in actual time just sixteen days have elapsed from the evening I first met consultant breast specialist, Muhamed Al-Dubaisi until today, the first seep of chemotherapy.

This feels fast, remarkably so in a country where medical repairs can take as long as domestic ones, the culture of the nine-month waiting list. Too quick, then? Well-meaning people say warningly, 'You're on the medical conveyor belt; have you stopped to explore other options?'

During the sixteen days there has been the diagnosis, the scrutiny to determine size and spread of the cancer, and there is my life – younger children to school, packed lunches, older children off on their long summer explorations, laundry and food-organizing, everybody else's various appointments, afternoons with Elon, laundry, ordinary family sicknesses and birthdays, and work.

Apparently though, I've left something out. The second opinion.

In London it is friends who've lost family to this illness who say, watch out for the doctors. From New York come phone calls: 'Are you coming over to Sloan Kettering? We can make you an appointment tonight, tomorrow, next week.' Sloan Kettering, New Yorkers tell you, is the only place for breast cancer: the shortest shot at saving your life. Elsewhere in the States, two of Anthony's clients independently proffer me my own team of specialists at Johns Hopkins.

People look askance when I dodge the question of the second opinion by saying, 'Uh, not yet, haven't had the time actually.' Eyebrows are raised further when they delve into my choice of specialist – how much research I did.

Cancer, I find out, is handled by teams. I couldn't have picked my team – surgeon Muhamed Al-Dubaisi, clinical oncologist Peter Ostler and radiologist Glenda Kaplan – in a less scientific way. I did exactly what my family doctor told me to do, which was to make an appointment with the first cancer specialist available. My only elaboration to this plan was to narrow my choice down to the first available at the hospital nearest home.

Mr Al-Dubaisi, who in this initial period I see most days, says he has no problems with second opinions. 'Many come to me for the second opinion,' he adds, the merest pressing together of the lips making it quite clear that for those who take this supermarket approach, this bulk-buying of medicine, he will be found in the section with the most select of products.

However, if I want a second opinion, he will happily give me a letter, but today, this minute, because in any event the chemotherapy must begin according to the timetable he has already laid out.

I remember Glenda Kaplan's dismissive shrug on the subject of second opinions, when she reported back on her colleagues' diagnosis of her sprained knee the morning I went to have a liver scan.

But the real problem as I see it is, how do you know who to ask for a second opinion? My sense of professions is that there are better people in each profession, but it takes some expertise to work out who they are. My previous experience of crisis was my divorce, during which I discovered, and reported as a journalist, that the so-called experts in the family law courts, the court welfare officers who question and make decisions about children in divorce cases, are ex-probation officers untrained in child issues. I left the family court very clear that it is crammed with bad lawyers, poor judges and shoddy experts. I could tell this because families, divorce and children are subjects I understand well. I am the expert on my children.

I couldn't begin to say which doctor might have a better understanding of my cancer; I don't even know what the broad medical issues are, let alone the fine distinctions.

I never get around to seeking that second opinion in these early days. Firstly, because I feel intuitively that I like my team; I trust them, and their concern for me. And second, because I don't feel I have the time it will take to work out which of the eminent experts really is the expert, without delaying my treatment.

I have the following conversation with Mr Al-Dubaisi.

'You know,' I ask, 'how you are always pressing to keep to a timetable, insisting that things must happen quickly, without delay? Is that medically crucial? Come on, it's a lump that's been sitting around for over three years by my reckoning; how much difference could a week here, a week there make?'

His answer is given with a grave face. 'Yes,' he says, 'it makes a difference. Not one week, but two, more than two, yes.'

So, sixteen days after being diagnosed, Anthony and I drop Elon at nursery in the pouring rain; Anthony's mother will pick him up for an afternoon of prime pampering. Sara-Jenny is putting highlights in her hair for the first time, a sixteen-year-old venture, more real to me than the chemotherapy, and I text her on the half-hour: 'How's it going now?'

The private wing of Mount Vernon is called Bishopswood. It looks like a motel, shades of beige, pink and green, and you are shown to your individual room with its small TV perched on the wall, and a lady comes and offers you a lunch menu. You don't see other patients like you do in the NHS parts of the hospital – private medicine meaning just what it says, it's a more private experience, with no wards. There are only spanking new newspapers delivered to your room by an orderly, no waiting rooms piled high with ancient copies of magazines, and the corridors don't echo like in the big old hospital buildings; they are lined with carpet, not ancient tiling.

I still don't really know what chemotherapy is. First comes the usual form filling – actually, all they want is the insurance authorization and, grimly, the next of kin. The thing about weeks of medical treatment is you begin to feel so dependent on the person squeezing the needle, on how they will make you feel, so I'm glad when today's nurse appears: Julie, Hollywood movie-star eyelashes, already speed-talking in her Scottish accent as she comes through the door, a little barmy, pretty, kind.

Peter Ostler, with his direct, unpatronizing look, follows her in and perches on the bed. He asks how I am, if I have any questions, and then pulls out a tape measure. I stand up so he can measure me against a wall. I have had a couple of appointments at which nurses and doctors have measured my height and weight, so that, as they've explained, they can correctly assess the chemotherapy dose. But today Peter Ostler looks confused as I back myself on to the wall, to stand tall for accuracy; he seems to be wondering where I'm going.

'Uh, no, not you – your breast,' his research assistant says.

'Oh,' I say, 'you're going to measure my breast. With a tape measure.'

In fact, it's the lump, which goes down in the notes as seven and a half centimetres by seven.

Two more hours, channel-hopping on the TV, texting the kids. We've brought a laptop with us, downloaded with the latest series of Larry David's *Curb Your Enthusiasm*, because I loved the couple of episodes I've already seen. We also have the two series of *24* that we resolutely missed, after the first hijacked our life. It's a standing joke in our house that I won't watch any more Jack Bauer with Anthony, though he keeps stockpiling the series on DVD as they come out. 'I don't have whole weeks to spend being exhausted because I had to stay up all night watching just one more episode,' I say plaintively. 'That awful sensation, you're just falling asleep, desperate for sleep actually, and then there's some action scene that completely jerks you awake again.'

'Dina does *24* like it's some kind of extreme sport,' Anthony's daughter Chloë chortles. But now, we have this sense that there will be acres of chemotherapy hours to fill, and we have come prepared. The idea is not to even notice the chemotherapy.

Finally, at one-thirty, three hours after we got here this morning, Julie flies in carrying a blue tray. She wraps a warming cushion round my right arm – 'Gets the veins up,' she says – and then begins the process of injecting the cannula – a needle through which she will take blood and drip the chemotherapy into my veins. Bending over to concentrate, though, she makes some awkward movement, and her back goes into a spasm, just as she puts the needle in. She practically crawls out of the room on all fours.

I only catch the end of this, Julie's retreating rear, because the top half of my body is twisted right away from the nursing action, on the principle that what you can't see hurts less, so I'm looking away, watching *Curb Your Enthusiasm* intently. But what was intended to be prime escapism is, today, making me flinch; nothing like needles for putting your emotions on edge. So what seemed brilliantly diverting just last night (some episode where Larry David refuses to be bound by funeral conventions and niceties) is now Larry David's grotesque trampling over everybody else. It's as if all the emotional energy I'm using to avoid feeling the pinprick of the needle is channelled into a hyper-alertness towards the feelings of the made-up characters on the laptop screen.

Like an extra see-through finger, a little plastic tube has grown into the vein on my right hand. This is the cannula, and all the medicine will go in through it.

Julie comes back – slightly stooped but smiling – carrying one of those huge, old-fashioned shower hats you'd see on some creaking body in a down-market soap opera, but this bit of headgear is so cold it's emanating icy smoke, a halo of visible chill. I've heard about the cold cap; it's a device that's supposed to stop your hair falling out. A number of people have said to me that I should make sure to ask for a cold cap if I'm not automatically offered one. Julie doesn't ask me, she just brings it in. 'If you don't get on wi' it, we'll take it off,' Julie says. Freezing cold from the end of the bed, once on my head it's like going under very cold water, or being out on a mountain, skiing. Julie has wrapped cotton wool around my ears and neck to protect them from the cold and folds a warm towel around my shoulders.

Finally the chemotherapy, liquid in a plastic bag that

hangs suspended from what looks like a music stand, like a very old man's head, bent over his cane. The Adriamycin and Cyclophosphamide is raspberry-coloured, and Julie has to stand next to the bed physically squeezing it into my veins, supervising each drop that enters me, because if any escapes into the bloodstream it will cause damage. 'It's a beautiful colour,' Anthony says.

'Aye, I like this one,' Julie says. 'I don't like the purple one, it looks unnatural going in. Red seems more right for the body.'

'I can feel it,' I say. There's a scratching under my skin.

'Some say it's like rats crawling up,' Julie says.

Forty-five minutes later, it's over. My nose is running, from the cold cap I guess, though maybe it's a chemotherapy side effect. I slip the soaps from the bathroom into my handbag, acting like I'm on a minibreak in some metropolitan city hotel, and off we go.

Back home people have brought whole meals in foil dishes and plastic containers. I invite Elly and her five children to stay and share the copious amounts of food, and we all eat out in the garden. Paper plates, no clearing up, no preparation. Elly's brought cherries, blueberries and raspberries, which feel like what's needed, fresh, appetite-stimulating colours. There are also email messages waiting for me, from Matt Seaton, whose first wife Ruth Picardie died of this. Matt, and others from the *Guardian*, write often, and the messages feel like a layer of protection, defending against the harshness of the treatments, and balancing out with unsolicited kindnesses the unsettling sensation of never knowing where the next medical shock is going to come from. I register a surprise in my mind at how much these missives from outside help.

This first chemotherapy late afternoon and evening I don't feel the overwhelming tiredness people seem to think I should be experiencing. I don't collapse into bed when we arrive home from hospital, but move into my usual late-afternoon mode. But it is like operating through a mild haze; a fogginess has settled over my mind, a woolly blanketing. There's a collection of tablets to take, which I do dutifully: small white ones, three a day for three days, then some longer, oval-shaped ones. I don't really know what they're for, except they're supposed to help in some way, with nausea I think. I put the packets in a bowl on the kitchen counter so I will remember them. I feel worse after I take them, but stick to the doses religiously.

Other things go awry. The day after the chemotherapy and it's non-uniform day at Nina's school, except I forget, and so does she, so I'm busy congratulating myself on dropping her off on time, and smartly pressed and lunch-boxed, before setting off on the longer amount of time it takes to settle Elon in at nursery for his two-hour morning session. I'm so pleased at the morning not going off the rails I don't notice what the other children at Nina's school are wearing. I return from dropping Elon at nursery, glad for these lingering school days of the summer term, the short few weeks until everyone is on holiday. But, like a split-screen film, Nina's bit of school drama has been picking up speed while I've been calmly reading extra stories to Elon to make sure he stays at nursery for the full morning, guaranteeing my couple of hours' break.

There's a message on the answering machine from Priscilla, the nanny my ex-husband employs: can she pick up Nina's denim skirt? When I get to the bottom of the tangled story it turns out that instead of taking the simple step of phoning me on my mobile, the school secretary has phoned Priscilla, 'so as not to bother Dina'. She has told Nina that 'Mummy's busy, it's her treatment today, we'll phone Daddy's house.'

The impudent and unhelpful kindness of others. Now Nina's in a state because she thinks, 'But Mummy doesn't have a treatment today – is there something she isn't telling me?' and she is mortified to be stuck in uniform while all around her are in their civilian gear.

I phone the school to say I will come and collect her so she can change – we live five minutes' walk, thirty seconds' drive, from the school. The secretary ums and ahs, and through the chemo haze I stay assertive and calm, saying, 'If you won't let me pick her up and bring her back to school, can you please call her to the phone so I can at least ask her which clothes she'd like me to bring in?'

I am glad to have stayed firm (school secretaries being as much hard work as doctors' receptionists) when I see Nina, and she is so relieved at having something to change into. She has been wearing the uniform for an hour and a half, every minute of which must have felt like being dressed like a traffic light. I curse the school, and their considerate reluctance to contact me as soon as she arrived this morning, and realized the mistake.

Now, there is just Anthony's birthday present to organize this morning. This rapidly descends into farce. Anthony's family are religious about birthdays, a no-expense-spared annual rite. One year I gave him a hand-made card and it was nearly second divorces all round.

The morning hijacked, there is no time to reach any of London's ritzier stores before picking Elon up from nursery. That means finding something in Hendon – not exactly destination shopping, unless your loved one craves a bagel for his birthday. Then I see a shop I have never noticed before. 'We fit car navigation systems,' the window boasts. It's perfect. Anthony has a terrible sense of direction and a new car he really loves. And they can fit it in one day. I phone Anthony to say my car's acting up, and can I use his tomorrow. Of course, he says, anything.

That afternoon, Nina can't stop saying how much she appreciated my bringing in her clothes. Over tea the other children all sympathize. Later, I lie on the carpet with her to colour in clouds for (yet another) show her class is putting on at school tomorrow, and I organize to meet Anne Fine at Kenwood.

Friday morning. I get Nina and Elon to school, and Anthony's car to the navigation-system fitters, before I'm back at Nina's school for the half-hour special assembly complete with clouds. Sara-Jenny is going to collect Elon from nursery for me, so I can interview Anne Fine without feeling pressured for time.

There was a time when a lot of the women in the upper reaches of the arts were like Fine – unreconstructed 1970s feminists, as she describes herself. She is already sitting, with her publicist Mary Byrne, in the Brew House café at Kenwood House when I arrive. It is a fresh-air find for me, Kenwood, a stately home ten minutes' drive away from our deeply unfashionable part of London.

I can get into my car and, on a weekday when the parking is easy, glide into the Kenwood House car park, walk along a leafy-covered gravel path, coming out into a massive expanse of green with a lake gleaming away in the distance. Smart left turn, past the white and cream pillared house, and down some steps into a high stone hall with wooden tables where the coffee's good, though the hot chocolate is watery.

Fine has cornflower-blue eyes, so she wears a lavender T-shirt under a blue crinkly jacket. Her hair is the softest grey. She sports her watch on her right wrist. All these things mark her out for me as a certain type of woman I met first in Fleet Street, a generation of career women, avant-garde in their time, but no longer. They learned to mark themselves out, give themselves distinctive trademarks (putting themselves in the hands of stylists if they couldn't do it themselves). Like the fledgling females at Nina's school, competing to be cool on a non-uniform day, women like Fine don't let it show, but they put some thought into what they wear.

Fine's generation of feminists mix authoritativeness with a package of characteristics designed to blunt the hard edge: a professed lack of professionalism ('I scribble anywhere,' she says), an airy claiming about being so hopeless with figures she doesn't even know how old she is (late fifties), nothing tough about their careerism, but all topped off with a firm, no-nonsense morality.

She tells me, straight off, just so we know where we are, how good she was at raising money for charity while she was children's laureate, the position bestowed every two years on one of the leading children's authors. 'A friend in America told me, the secret of raising money is to ask for it. So,' she continues, 'you do know Philip (Pullman), and Jackie (Wilson) and J. K. Rowling do have more than enough money. If someone like me calls, not a single one hesitates for a moment. I had £30,000 straight away.'

Equally straightforwardly, Fine says to me, of mastectomy: 'Well, I'd much rather lose a breast than one of anything else,' which actually turns out to be the most sensible, and indeed comforting, thing anybody has to say on the subject.

She was in her early twenties when her own mother contracted breast cancer, and underwent a range of treatments – 'mastectomy and other mysterious things'. Her mother didn't tell her what she was going through until afterwards. 'I thought it hurtful and extraordinary,' Fine says.

'Yes,' I agree. And I tell her how the doctors ask me for my family medical history, and I have to say I don't know it, that I don't have good relations with my family, but that I think my grandmother had breast cancer, and that I believe my mother had a hysterectomy for some condition or other, and that I did have a card from one of my sisters saying her doctor said she should let her siblings know about her colon cancer.

Fine listens to this rush of information kindly, non-judgemental. I don't know, before we meet, that I will end up talking to her about the breast cancer. I know that I want to carry on writing my children's author pages for the *Guardian*, that it is the kind of work I can do even if somewhat incapacitated. It is just a monthly commitment, more than manageable.

But, with Meg Rosoff still in my mind, and now Fine's open talking about her mother, it feels like the children's authors are becoming markers for the way ahead, the road that is this illness, like pebbles dropped by Hansel and Gretel. Maybe because, as in all the best children's stories, my parents are absent during this time of peril for me, or maybe because the children's authors – these keepers of the story-telling flame – are rounded with wisdom, or maybe just because my emotions are heightened with chemotherapy drugs, but it feels like I've tapped into a support network I didn't even know was out there.

When I leave Fine I feel stronger, a feeling compounded by further self-contentment as, back home after the interview, I check in the mirror and my hair is still intact. Yes! The rational approach to keeping my hair where it belongs – on my scalp – is working. I've done everything right: the short, sharp crop, the no-expense-spared wig, bandanna rehearsal runs (collecting the children from school in an assortment of vibrantly coloured scarves tied trendily, even though my hair is looking its best). Why, I even embraced the medically devised cold cap – these actions will forestall hair loss, I have been telling myself. How do I know? I know this, because I come from generations of Lithuanian Mitnagdim.

Amongst us Ashkenazi Jews – we who can carry a gene for breast cancer – there is a dividing line: Chassidim versus Mitnagdim. Chassidic Jews cornered the emotional; we Mitnagdim are the logicians. I grew up knowing that mine is a Judaism of rigorous thinking, demanding scepticism. Superstition belongs to the others. So I feel confident my hair will stay put – coming from the stock I do, it's just using my head. Act like your hair will fall out, and of course it won't. Otherwise posited as: 'inside every rationalist huddles a wild-eyed amulet-wearer facing cancer'.

As the day goes on, the wild-eyed, demented version of me pushes ever closer to the surface. By four o'clock the chap who is supposed to be putting the finishing touches to Anthony's whizzy new navigation system is phoning with excuses. By five, I realize I've made a terrible and very expensive mistake. Back early from work, Anthony walks around the corner with me to the auto shop. Bits of his car are lying all over the garage. Thank God I have cancer.

Meanwhile, it turns out the little white pills are appetite stimulants as well as sickness suppressants. So, starving and nauseous. Excellent combination.

This is where community really kicks in. Food arrives in a steady stream, almost intravenously. Anthony's old friends, Dennis and Gillian, bring gazpacho so fresh you can taste every vegetable. We all eat it for Friday-night dinner and for the next three days I eat nothing else.

Over the weekend there are many guests. So many callers have come in with food, I find myself inviting others to share it with abandon. Big mistake. By Sunday night, after clearing away for the nineteenth time, I'm in bed with every limb trembling. I have weird dreams all night long, and keep waking up feeling frightened. It reminds me of films I've seen where they show the characters lying in bed trembling as they withdraw from drugs or alcohol. I've got the DTs, I tell myself.

There's a metallic taste in my mouth, and a craving for healthy foods and spa treatments, seaweed and skin-brushing and seeds. Instead of which, I'm harassing Sara-Jenny about exactly what her plans are over the summer. By Tuesday morning I find myself just sitting at the kitchen table, holding myself very still, as breakfast happens around me.

'Anthony,' I say, 'I need you to do the baby, please.' We all call Elon the 'baby', though his third birthday is just weeks away. The children make their own lunches, and Anthony does the school run in my car because his new blue Saab, the first car he has ever loved owning, is still beached in the drive of the 'latest technology CD and sat-nav systems' store so conveniently close to us, just five minutes' walk away, if that.

All I have to do is interview Robert Winston (I'm stacking up children's authors these first weeks, so I have a store of taped interviews in case it becomes harder to see people over the next few months). Winston, a life peer and one of the most famous fertility doctors, has an easy way of explaining science that makes him a natural for television documentaries (not to mention a pronounced resemblance to Albert Einstein). Somewhere, on the side, he's written a book for children about the human body, *What Makes Me Me?* which is the only reference book left lying around our kitchen that I've seen the children pick up. This immediately triggers my journalist's quivering nose, because, these days, reference books are no-interest zones for the kids, every school assignment being just a click on the Internet – but Winston's book has, ingeniously, built-in personality quizzes.

Originally insisting I do the interview at his hospital between his other meetings, on the basis that he has 'no free time until November', when I phone his secretary to say I've just had chemotherapy and so I think I'm not supposed to go into hospitals because of the increased risk of infection (which belief turns out to be nonsense, in fact, when I double-check with my oncologist), Lord Winston replies within minutes that it will be fine for me to see him at his home, ten minutes' drive away from where I live. Opening the door himself, he turns out to be not only solicitous, but also a gadget boffin, making me a great coffee for about ten minutes using a steam engine, I think – something that takes a certain amount of cranking, anyhow, and produces huge amounts of white, puffing stuff. He knows all about navigation systems: 'Ah yes,' he says, 'they're not all that developed yet.'

∞

The next few days are muggy, threatening the end of July and the closing of the school year. My limbs feel trembly all week, juddering like a car engine dying. I keep trying to take naps but it's all punctuated by relentless phone hassles with the sat-nav people.

Walking to collect Elon from nursery I come back soaked in sweat – still over-tired. Back home, I change and try very hard to look cool, calm and, above all, wholly rational, while I walk with Elon round the corner to continue negotiations at the auto store about how they will now remove the super-duper in-car navigation system, which has completely mucked up the music system and the crucial hands-free phone system, from Anthony's car.

Previous discussions with the fitter have not gone well. Predictably, today ends with me shrieking, and him snapping, 'Keep your hair on, lady.'

Eventually they take our threats of suing seriously – 'I hear you're a very important lawyer,' the owner says to Anthony – and it only takes forty-five minutes to put the car back together again and refund my money. A few days late, I buy Anthony a birthday iPod.

5. The Summer of Change

Throwing out a pineapple skin I brush the inside of my wrist lightly with the jagged edge. It's such a brief encounter, and soft, like a dandelion clock. But a second later a dull red bruise is spreading across the veined area, before my eyes. 'Huh?' I hear myself say.

One week after the first chemotherapy and I'm a walking biology lesson, so interesting I could qualify for a mention in a Robert Winston tome.

'Do you know how they discovered this treatment?' Julie, the chemo nurse, asked, chattily, the day she stood by my bed putting in the drugs. 'After the war, they did autopsies on mustard-gas victims, discovered the gas had stopped bone-marrow growth, and the bodies had low blood-cell counts, so some bright spark figured they could use the same stuff to stop cancer cells growing.'

And the effect of this particularly nasty and debilitating First World War poison on me, circa 2005? Well, white blood cells are your line of resistance against the outside world. Chemotherapy, in its race to kill off the mad, mutating cancer cells, attacks the good guys along with the bad.

When your white cells are down, the merest graze ends up looking like you just took a hammer to yourself.

The fatigue is still low-grade, ditto the nausea. It is, as I keep saying to everyone who asks, very like being pregnant, if you throw in the exhaustion of the years after giving birth.

But the post-chemotherapy weariness has this edge to it – if I push things too far, I end up in bed at night with trembling limbs and a racing heart. It's an anxiety that feels like a druggy reaction.

Anthony and I go to bed early these nights, watching DVDs. We watch the episode of *Sex and the City* where Samantha has chemotherapy. She sits in a thickly padded lounger, controls to ease her back and forth, like a very luxurious dentist's chair, sucking ice lollies with her friends. I remember catching this bit before, when it was on television for the first time, and barely taking in the details – it couldn't have had less to do with us. Now, I'm gazing in wonder at the American-style 'chemo-lounge'.

My eyes are drooping, heavy-lidded, when I realize Anthony is crying as Samantha shaves off her hair on the screen. I sit up and catch Rudolf Nureyev, as Carrie's boyfriend, saying doesn't she realize Samantha could die? It doesn't even occur to me that dying is a possibility. As I fall into a disturbed sleep I'm thinking, 'Don't suppose losing a breast would seem all that important if I thought I might die from this . . .'

Deeper into this night of fitful sleep, the house silent, Anthony motionless, my mind racing with dreams, my girls at their father, and Anthony's children at their mother, I wander from room to room like Goldilocks, trying out every bed in the house, seeking peace. Ours is the quietest room by far, I realize, the least invaded by traffic, yet we sleep the least.

Underneath all the symptoms, and maybe this is the drug anxiety again, I feel an unease that because I'm still functioning pretty normally – I'm not laid up, it's nothing like the dread stuff intimated by people's shocked faces when they hear the word chemotherapy – it can't be working. I check and can't see any sign that the lump is shrinking at all yet. It feels like a hard, heavy metal plate in my sad, soft breast.

So, when they appear, I welcome the second wave of distorted bodily functions. As the nausea settles, diarrhoea and mouth ulcers take over – ah, that explains the ice lollies then – like pit stops the drug is taking on its route round my body. The diarrhoea's fine, because it makes swift work of the weight I've put on from the steroids they give you to counter sickness; and the mouth ulcers get treated by a bright green wash called Difflam, which becomes my drink of choice for a number of days.

Speaking of which, after being happily weaned on to chocolate milk in a bottle, suddenly Elon has started asking for breast milk again. I tell him my breasts are still there, but there's no more 'meee' – his word for breast milk. 'But I just like "meee",' he says, 'I only want "meee".' He walks off with a sad face.

There is a sense, in our house, of changes, of things shifting. Today is the last day of the summer term. Elon, the August baby, marches proudly into nursery with birthday-party invitations, moving his arms like train pistons as he goes happily into the room, because Nina has hand-crafted his invitations to read, 'chug along to Elon's party . . .'

We have to decide what to do with Elon this coming academic year. After a term sampling a few morning hours in a nursery, Elon is due to start kindergarten at the primary school he will attend. But should we shift him from his ideal, three-hour nursery mornings – six children, two loving adults – into the bigger arena of junior school, when, because he is an August-born child, we could hold him back a year, which would mean he stays in nursery until all my treatment is over?

I have never been away from him overnight, and – though he is my fourth child – I'm bone-shakingly anxious about how he will react during the week I need to be in hospital for surgery.

All I want now, during this crisis, is to keep everything as routine for Elon as possible, and not subject him to any unnecessary changes. I know the surgery will be in the autumn – chemotherapy is every three weeks, I am having four rounds before surgery, so that takes us to October or thereabouts. This means if we do take Elon out of the nursery and move him to the primary school for kindergarten, he will have just begun in a whole new environment when I suddenly disappear to hospital for a week. When Nina was his age I was separating from her father – it doesn't take me all that long to understand that the breast cancer is only part of why this decision about Elon seems so huge. In a badly managed school, where her anxieties from home were compounded by poor emotional support in the classroom, Nina's pain from those days lives with me still. Moreover, it's not just a new school to Elon; Anthony and I are trying a school for Elon that none of our other children has ever attended.

No surprise, then, that the day we visit the kindergarten is only the second time in his life that Elon acts up (the first was when he had to come with me to an interview with Bianca Jagger, she transcendentally calm in pale-pink linen pyjamas, he a screaming, spewing mass of baby). In the airy, toy-filled room, he clings on to me, crying when anybody approaches him. 'He's really not like this,' I say with a spitting, furious toddler choking my neck. My bright, happy boy is a changed creature. The kindergarten head is relaxed, and equally firm that her view is he should transfer as originally planned, so he begins school with the rest of his age group, although at the tail end.

The summer of change. There are too many days now that I don't recognize myself. I hear my voice screaming at Sara-Jenny, in a way I've never sounded before. 'Either you tell me exactly what your plans are, or I'm cancelling your ticket!' Even as I shriek at her over the stairs I'm shocked by the rage issuing from my mouth. It's not what I'm saying, it's the pitch of it. A mad, foaming fury.

Sara-Jenny looks white, mutinous, at the bottom of the staircase. I go back into my room, sit on the bed shaking, and can feel the heat rising through my body. I touch my cheeks and they're red hot.

Somewhere along the way I've read that chemotherapy can start the menopause. I can't even say when the hot flushes started – I've just vaguely noticed that, from always being cold, these days I'm periodically suffused with heat.

I keep trying to imagine what losing a breast will be like. This right breast is going to be cut away, I say to myself, trying to get some sense of the reality of it. In my life I have lost daily contact with my children. Second Thursdays they go to their father for a long weekend. Though I spent months discussing the children's arrangements before implementing them, the words were meaningless. I did not understand the loss until the day it happened. When I describe it, I say it was like a piece of my body had been hacked out.

It's Tisha B'av, the ninth day of the Hebrew month of Av, a culmination of a three-week period of mourning for Jews. The twenty-four-hour fast is considered the saddest day in the Jewish calendar, commemorating the destruction of both the first and second Temples, both destroyed on the ninth of Av (the first by the Babylonians in 586 BC, the second by the Romans in 70 AD).

One of the first questions I had asked Mr Al-Dubaisi, as I tried to piece my way through this new terrain, was, 'Can I fast?'

'Do you fast like us?' he said, smiling. 'Though it's many years since I've fasted – but you know, Ramadan?'

'No,' Anthony interjected, anxiously. 'Moslems eat at nightfall, don't they; some of the Jewish fasts are twenty-four hours long, and there is no drinking.' Anthony, lawyer that he is, ends with what he considers to be the clincher.

'Mm, it's fine,' Mr Al-Dubaisi came back. 'No problem. Just carry on as you would normally.'

'What, somersaults, everything?' I asked. Back in May, that time pre-breast cancer, I enrolled in an adult gym class at Hendon Leisure Centre. For years the children have been going to gym there, it's one of Hendon's specialities, and the children's gym classes are so overbooked you have to be prepared to get up at five to join a line if you want to secure a child a place.

When I had signed up for myself I said my ambition was to do a cartwheel, and the man behind me in the queue said it takes two years, but that I would get there. I made two of the classes before my diagnosis of breast cancer. There is one other woman in the class at about the same level of (non-) gymnastics as I am; but otherwise the class is a group of twenty-somethings who were born doing back-flips.

The sessions are two hours long, and take place on Sunday afternoons from 5 p.m. Booking myself into a class at tea-time on a Sunday was an acknowledgement of Elon's moving out of infancy; my not being needed every second any more, a handing over to his dad for two hours on a weekend. I had a sense of reclaiming my life, of Elon beginning to start independent existence.

The classes are tough. The first hour, most of which I spend checking the clock, is an aerobic work-out – ninety-seven different ways of running round the slightly bouncy, foot-smelling floor of the gym. Then you start the gymnastics, working on the handstand, the somersault, the backwards somersault and, astonishingly, the hanging from two round hoops on a bar and swinging over a pit filled with foam blocks. It takes remarkably little of this (and the teacher pulls out a specially padded giant blue mattress for me to attempt handstands against by the second of those lessons) before I decide that adult gymnastics doesn't come under the category of 'normal carrying on' while undergoing chemotherapy.

Fasting, on the other hand, is fine. In fact, this Tisha b'Av is a lot easier than the fasting this time last year when Elon was still a hungry breast-feeder. I can remember the hot summer day, and the craving for water which I quenched by splashing my face incessantly from the tap.

This Tisha B'Av Elon climbs on to my lap and sticks his face down my shirt. 'Hee-hee, Mummy, one of your sides is sticking out.'

Bizarrely, with the chemotherapy, the right breast has started to droop oddly over my bra – I don't know if this is the effect of the drug on the lump within. I tell Elon there is no 'meee' in the breast any more, and then I say briskly, 'OK, enough now, let's get you a drink,' a request with which he is, as these transforming months go on, increasingly happy to acquiesce. I still marvel a bit at how you can tell a child 'no more milk' and that's it. We are settling into these new patterns.

And then my hair starts to fall from my head. Like being at a bad hairdresser, it is round my neck, in my eyes, gently drifting down my face, entwined in my fingers every time I put hand to face.

Elon wakes in the night and I lay my cheek close against his, my tried and tested soothing measure; it works in a matter of seconds, this primal stroking of head to head, until he calms and sleeps again. I fall back into my own bed, only to be jerked back awake again almost instantly. Elon is sitting straight up against his pillow, twisting uncomfortably, his mouth writhing, as he calls: 'Mummy, Mummy, I've got hair in my mouth.'

It's all over my pillow too. Just single hairs, but every time I open my eyes I see a strand in front of me. There is a frizzing sensation where hair meets scalp, as if I've had a terrible 70s perm, and each hair has been burned at the root. In the morning I don't touch my head, but I go to the mirror to stand and stare. I'm blearily surprised at how much hair I still have.

I take a Sunday out, leaving Anthony with the children. I'm on the train to Newcastle to interview Eva Ibbotson, author of a childhood classic, *Journey to the River Sea*. The chemotherapy-induced diarrhoea and mouth ulcers have really settled in now. I thank God that King's Cross railway station has clean toilets, though you have to pay for them, and my need is almost too urgent for the requisite fumbling to find coins for the slots. I upgrade myself to First Class on the train, and do the mouth ulcers no favour by settling back with a packet of salt-and-vinegar crisps. I think there's a kind of bloody-mindedness about the way I finish the whole bag.

Then I pick up an abrupt message on my mobile from Eva Ibbotson. 'I hope you can get lunch on the train.'

I phone her to reassure her about lunch. 'Of course I don't need feeding,' I say. She tells me she's had her grandchildren all weekend, and they've cleaned her out, and that because she is so old herself, she doesn't actually eat.

I know Ibbotson suffers from lupus, but I don't actually know what that is. When I get to her house, in a quiet, shady corner of Newcastle called Jesmond, the door is opened by one of her sons. Up a grand staircase, and in a beautiful, sun-filled, peacock-blue room, with a mantelpiece laden with photos, she's sitting very upright in a wing-backed chair. There's a cube on the mantelpiece imprinted with the words: WRITER'S BLOCK. She has grey hair and brown-grey eyes, and she's wearing a grey polo neck under a trouser suit.

I come in and sit down, and we both reach for water. I notice we're both dribbling, not quite in control of our dry mouths. 'I don't suppose you know abut illness,' she says, beadily.

'Yes, I do!' I counter. 'I'm having chemo at the moment – I have breast cancer – I'm pretty sick from it too, can't eat a thing – no need for lunch!'

Oh, her expression says, trumped. With that, we are friends, another pebble shining in the moonlight.

Hours into what becomes a long, chatty afternoon, sipping our waters, and I'm easily discussing intimate physical details with an older woman I've never met before. It is becoming a part of this story.

Ibbotson knows about families. Her father, it emerges, a refugee from Nazi Germany, was one of the first scientists to work with sperm donation. In those early, unregulated days, the sperm pioneers used their own semen rather than relying on canvassing volunteers. Eva has half-siblings all over the world.

On the train home, I scribble notes and impressions from the interview, and when I look back from the train window to the page on the table before me there's a hair, just one, foetally curled, the way I sleep.

6. Losing It

From: 'Dina Rabinovitch' Dina_Rabinovitch@yahoo.co.uk
To: 'Ian Katz' Ian.Katz@guardian.co.uk
Subject: hair

Dear Ian – if you pick this up, tragically my hair has started coming out . . . tho' Anthony's putting up with comments about, at least Dina's hair isn't disappearing as fast as his . . . but anyhow, it's certainly killing me . . . so, if at all possible, can we do photos before it gets worse . . . ?
Best, Dina

The week I am diagnosed I email Becky Gardiner at the *Guardian* (an editor for whom I wrote a column about being a mother who helps out at school) to tell her I'm ill, and that I'd like to write about it, in a column describing this illness, this treatment. I want the column to run in the main newspaper, on what's called the op-ed page, the one facing the editorials, the leader columns, the heavyweight opinion-forming page. But the opinion-page editor will only agree to run one piece a month op-ed, and neither Becky nor I think that will be enough to establish it as a regular feature.

'If one in nine men were losing their penises, you can bet this'd be an op-ed story,' I say to Becky. 'In fact, it'd be a front-page story. Daily.'

Ian Katz is on the phone almost within minutes of my

first negotiations about the column, saying he wants it for G2, the *Guardian*'s features section, and that I will not regret it – 'if you see our statistics you'll know that G2 is by far the best-read section of the paper'. Then, later that week, he says, 'Well, if you want to go with me, you're going to have to let me know by the end of today. I'm going on holiday and this is the last day to take the decision about this kind of column.'

A mix of empathy and brisk negotiation, Ian's a bracing outside person during these first post-chemotherapy weeks. We firm up how the column will run, that it will start in the first week of September and then – a judgement by me about what I can commit to given the chemotherapy schedule – run fortnightly after that. Ian says they'll need to take some pictures, and I hang up forgetting to say, 'before my hair falls out'. So now, as my hair starts to come out of my head, I email him.

'Poor you,' he writes back, 'hang in . . .'

The mouth ulcers and the diarrhoea fade, and Sara-Jenny leaves for Israel, the days in the run-up to her trip a fog of last-minute shopping. The three weeks between chemotherapy treatments are now pockets of time into which life is slotted. We will head to Cornwall later this summer with some of the children at least, slotting in the vacation between everybody's camp commitments, their other parents and cancer treatment. I negotiate with Peter Ostler, leaving a message with his secretary to ask whether my treatment dates can be flexible at all. 'A day either side doesn't matter,' he replies, 'but there's some evidence that going over three weeks is not beneficial.'

'Not a read-story,' Elon says that night, 'I want a tell-story.' OK. That means making one up; what should it be about? 'Umm, a bicycle and Mummy's hair.'

This permeates the children more than I realize. Although my hair's been falling out for a few days now, there is still so much on my head I didn't think Elon had noticed anything. But he has heard the talk, obviously. 'It looks normal, just thin,' Nina says, coming downstairs one morning, and putting her arms around me. 'I didn't know how it would fall out,' she adds. I put fingers to my head, and whole tresses come away. But there's still a lot to go.

It's Elon's third birthday. The day starts the way all days start now, cleaning the hair out of the floor of our shower. How much hair I still have. I'm physically conscious of the contact between my hair and my scalp; it feels as if the hair is brittle and that's why it's dropping off, but when I see it on my fingers, hold the fallen hair on my hand, it's not sizzled and burned, as I imagine, it's still sleek and silky – but it is so constant, this incessant drifting-down. Drifts of hair pile up on the newly tiled bathroom floor.

Bizarrely, one of the things that gets done during this summer of chemotherapy is work on the house. So the splattered bathroom carpet we inherited is now cool green tiles. My mind is sluggish, but it's running at just the right speed for dealing with builders, i.e. cups of tea and not minding how long anything takes because my world has slowed down so much anyhow. And I bless the new floor, from which the hair sweeps so smoothly.

We make fairy cakes for the party this afternoon.

Green, pink, blue and yellow icing goes everywhere. The kitchen looks like something created by Jackson Pollock, on acid. But the chemotherapy slow-mindedness is also just right for looking after small children; my pace of living is about the same as Elon's now, so when he wants to measure the flour, I'm not my former impatient self. However long things take is fine, because that's how slow I am now. The mess lies all around, and I'm not whirling around like a dervish cleaning, I'm taking it easy.

'Ugh, eyelash,' Marganit says, looking down at yellow icing whirls. No, not eyelash, it's hair, of course. My hair.

'Give me a hug,' Elon says at bedtime.

'Sure,' I say, holding him at arm's width, 'but my naughty hair keeps falling out, I don't want it to get in your mouth.'

'Foot hug, then,' Elon says, chuckling.

My second chemotherapy session and Peter Ostler, wearing his summer white trousers, checked shirt and red tie, looks at my head and says, 'See, nobody would know you're having treatment.' I stare back at him in disbelief; my hair is thin, dry and woolly. Dr Ostler says not to touch it too much. I'm already covering it every day with a bandanna, though I don't have the right big-hoop earrings yet. Also I have to wear the bandanna further down my forehead, I realize, from star-gazing in *Hello* magazine.

Round Hendon, where so many women wear scarves over their hair for religious Jewish reasons, I want to look edgy, fashionable, not covered. It doesn't entirely work, though – the first time I go to the supermarket bandanna-ed, the (non-Jewish but local) woman on the till who sees me more than most friends, says, 'Oh, have you become more orthodox?' But at Elon's birthday party, none of the mothers mention my bandanna or ask if there's a reason I'm wearing it. For weeks now I've worn a bandanna off and on.

How fast the adjustments to new realities come. Medically, I already have a new obsession. Dr Ostler measures the lump this second session, and it is smaller, by one centimetre. The thought that's starting to occupy me is if the chemotherapy shrinks the tumour, why then do I need a mastectomy rather than a lumpectomy? Don't doctors have a history of doing too much that is unnecessary to women? I don't raise it yet; it's just beginning to fester.

Meanwhile, Dr Ostler is chatting, telling me the results of my latest tests. My tumour is oestrogen negative. It is a type known as Her-2 positive. Cancer tumours come in a bewildering array of varieties, I am starting to learn. That's one of the reasons they're so hard to cure; the cells mutate for numerous different reasons, triggered by hordes of factors.

'Oestrogen positive is the good kind, isn't it?' I say.

'Well, we can treat oestrogen-positive ones with certain drugs,' he says, 'but don't think you'd rather have that type, because there are so many variables.' One of the issues around my sort of tumour may be whether to remove the ovaries – he says this tentatively – although, he adds, the latest research seems to indicate that taking out ovaries isn't all that helpful. 'The findings are reported twice a year,' he says, 'so the next conference will be in time for you.'

But though the tumour is oestrogen and progesterone negative, Ostler says, my team are still anxious that I shouldn't have hormones sloshing around my body. I'll probably keep my ovaries, but I'm going to have to change my form of contraception, currently a coil with added hormones. He tells me he's already spoken to my family doctor about removing it. We will have to use contraception, he says, because any question of being pregnant while on chemotherapy needs to be covered, but the only acceptable method for now (as far as the doctors are concerned, anyhow) is condoms. Sitting in the corner of the room, Anthony grimaces.

'Very mobile lymph node,' Dr Ostler adds, moving on briskly and using his ruler under my arm now.

'But that is good, isn't it?' I say.

'Not when you're trying to measure it,' he answers.

A nurse – not Julie, whose back problems have flared up – comes in with the cold cap. I tell Dr Ostler I've heard some people won't wear one, to make sure the drugs reach everywhere in the body. 'That,' says my oncologist, 'would only apply to about two per cent of women who have a cancer that's spread to other organs, not one this local. But somebody is told something like that, then it filters down to everyone. The Internet,' he says, returning to one of his favourite themes, 'is not the best place to find information. Well, all except the few recognized sites, like Bacup, those are the only ones to read. Really, don't go looking round the Net,' he adds, a doctor working with experimental drugs, looking askance at another area of the newest technology.

The centre parting of my hair is so painfully bare that

I flinch when I see it. Still, I figure I'll give the cold cap one last fling. 'Oh, hair's coming out,' the nurse says as she adjusts the shower-cap-like device. 'Have you got a wig?'

Various email miscommunications mean that the *Guardian* photographer is coming to take photographs the day after this second chemotherapy, not a time guaranteed to display my best angles. Elon and Nina are both doing a day camp for this week, Nina ecstatically mucking out stables and riding horses – equestrian life is another surprising Hendon fact: we have not one, but two stables within easy reach – and Elon occupied with playgroup activities for the mornings. Anthony drops them off today and I start fretting about my hair. I pile conditioner into it to try and get rid of the frizziness, which doesn't work. Instead, when I rinse off the conditioner, whole hanks of hair come off. By the time the photographer arrives, much later on that afternoon, I'm in a bandanna, and on my third dose of the mood-boosting steroids the doctors give you to counter the effects of the chemotherapy, and Nina and Elon are both at a high pitch of overexhaustion. On the photographer's digital screen this translates into riotous scenes of happy family life. It is a cliché of this illness – photographs of women smiling brightly through adversity.

I keep trying to arrange a time with Sarah, my hairdresser, to cut my hair off completely, but she can't do it for a few days. It's too personal a moment to walk into a strange salon, or even to go to the hairdressers' where Sarah works and let somebody else cut the rest of my hair off. So I sit out the few days, but my hair deteriorates horribly and each day I'm waiting feels like a month. The hair doesn't just come out, leaving behind a smooth scalp; it hangs from my head in clumps and hunks, becoming matted in places, scarily absent elsewhere on my scalp. I look deranged, wild. It is the worst week. When I do finally meet up with Sarah to have it all cut off, she looks shocked at the state it's in. I should have cut it off much, much sooner in this hot, humid summer.

The children look white when I come back home after I finally see Sarah for a buzz-cut. All except the youngest, that is. Elon is wreathed in chuckles: 'Ha, ha, look at Mummy,' he chortles as he brushes his fingers delightedly through the soft fuzz left on my scalp.

That night Nina is crying softly in the bathroom. When I come in and sit down next to her, she blurts out that her own hair is thinning, and that it's my fault, because I make her wash it too often.

7. Of Blokes and Boobs

'I'm a bloke,' Peter Ostler says, using the technical terminology, 'so I can't really say, but in my opinion you're better off without it.' He's talking, naturally, about my breast.

The summer has swept past. Elon, Marganit, Nina and I have tales of being caught in the Boscastle floods – North Cornwall's biggest ever rescue operation according to the news – on a day when Anthony drove back to London from Cornwall to fetch Chloë and Theo, and one week on, I am safely back in hospital having my third chemotherapy treatment.

The dread increases with each treatment. The chemotherapy has a pattern: leaden fatigue in the days immediately after each dose, then the nausea and other symptoms hit, and finally everything recedes and I forget feeling bad. But the treatment comes round again relentlessly. When the chemo subsides and you feel fine for a few days you don't even really notice how well you're feeling, until another treatment looms. A major factor in the dread is the sick anticipation of which nurse will be putting in the needle, and how smoothly, or otherwise, that insertion will happen. Today, it's the senior sister. 'Oh, tough, this,' she says as she puts in her needle. I curdle inwardly and smile thinly back at her.

She breezily asks me if I use the cold cap, looking down at her notes. Then, looking up, she says, 'Oh, no point, I see you've lost your hair.'

She goes off to see if the chemotherapy is 'off hold' – the terminology they use to mean that the drug is ready to be infused. Each dose, made up to each patient's specifications, is kept on hold until the doctor says the patient is well enough to take the medicine. If it's taken off hold, and then the patient isn't fit enough to have the dose, the drug would have to be thrown away.

Dr Ostler is, I think, the youngest of the specialists looking after me. Each chemotherapy treatment he appears, in a flurry of nurses and research assistants, and perches on the bed to answer questions, leaving the small medical fry dotted against the walls, clipboards poised, like captured butterflies. He's ambitious, I think, so if I tell him I've heard about someone who has died of this disease, he says, 'Not a patient of mine?' with a kind of possessiveness of good outcomes for his patients.

These ten-minute chats pre-chemotherapy (£830.92 worth of A C) bill at £380 a time, which doesn't reflect their value. A friend whose teenage daughter is hospitalized for months says she is still waiting for just one of her daughter's doctors to sit on the bed, rather than stand at the end, looking down.

I ask Dr Ostler if it's true that, as the general perception has it, there is more breast cancer than there used to be in women my age. 'It's still low,' he replies, 'about fifteen per hundred, but it does feel like it's increasing. Although maybe it just didn't used to be polite to tell someone they had cancer,' he adds, with a little smile for the bad old days before doctors perched on beds.

He doesn't have pat answers; he thinks while he speaks. So, he continues, 'I have a sense that I'm seeing more women my own age,' he says, 'but possibly that's because the over-seventies we see once, the treatment is routine. But someone like you I will see much more, because we are concerned to get the effects of the treatment as right as possible for your stage of life.'

What does he think about giving up dairy products? 'Yes,' he sighs, 'my colleagues are always sending me the data. But there's the loss of calcium, and the dangers of osteoporosis. One of my patients stopped having chemotherapy and lives on carrots – she's orange now. I wouldn't like to be orange.'

How about weekly chemotherapy, as practised in the States, as opposed to the fortnightly or three-weekly cycles on this side of the Atlantic? 'Ah,' he says, with a you've-been-cruising-the-Net-again expression, 'it's true that so far the results look very good, but we know that over the course of a study those results can change. So, over here, we tend to wait.

'Also,' he says, 'I suppose we in Europe are somewhat cynical, because these drugs are so very expensive, we think American oncologists are just considering how much money they can make.' Then, a little abashed, he adds, 'Of course, you always get that kind of talk this side of the ocean.'

And so to mastectomy. Oncologically better, he says.

'Still, if you tell me you really, really want to keep the breast, then . . .' and he tails off.

This is called, as I believe the correct bloke terminology would have it, throwing me a googly. Mr Al-Dubaisi has never spoken in any terms other than mastectomy – removing the lump alone, rather than the whole breast, has not once figured in any of the times we have sat, contemplating the ins and outs of this disease, across a desk from him. But now the oncologist is looking at me with compassion, and also an urging, it seems to me, to take control of this process.

In my mind I can hear the global breast-cancer community cheering. Read the books – from Jane Plant's *Your Life in Your Hands* to *Breast Cancer for Dummies* – and surf the Internet sites, and it's all about information, this assumption that involving yourself in your healthcare, this very act of gathering knowledge is empowering and therefore (somehow) beneficial to the outcome, to saving your life from cancer. The crux of it seems to be that being involved in one's own medical decision-taking makes the patient feel more positive about the course of treatment. And 'positive' is the holiest cancer mantra of them all. (Although, not, let it be said, positive in the sense of saying yes; because 'pleasers' you know, are so susceptible to cancer, they qualify as tumour magnets.)

The closet cancer psychologists are forever telling me that 'being positive is really good'. They tell me my frequent smiling is 'excellent'. How, I wonder, can my mood – which depends mainly on what I weigh, actually – affect the deadliness with which my cells are dividing?

And then, from the other side, come the mood-gaugers who apparently are not beneficiaries of my beauteous smiles. A mother from Nina's school informs me about 'expelling anger'. 'Someone like me,' she says, 'would never get cancer, because I'm always blabbing, but you, you're very intellectual, terribly controlled, you must let your feelings out.'

Now, with only one more chemotherapy session to go before the planned operation, my oncologist, whose opinions I do value, seems to be agreeing with the books: have some influence over the course of your treatment; what is 'oncologically best' may not be the whole picture.

On the way home I speak to Sara-Jenny, still in Israel, but coming home in a few days. She has, she tells me, spoken to her grandparents, my mother and father, and has told them about the cancer. Not that day, but the next, I phone them myself, tell them I'm fine. My mother says that her mother died of breast cancer. 'Didn't you know?' she asks me.

The afternoon before Rosh Hashana, the Jewish New Year, I have the last of this first set of four chemotherapy treatments. When it's over I feel unexpectedly happy, although until the sense of relief and freedom washes over me I hadn't even realized I was counting the days. Peter Ostler appears during the treatment and says straight away, 'I read your piece.' The column about this breast cancer, 'The Enemy Within', has just started running in the *Guardian*. There's an odd time-lag: here I am, finished a huge, first stage of the treatment, and in 'newspaper time' I have only just been diagnosed.

'Which one did you read?' I ask him. 'First or second?'

'Oh, there's another one?' he says.

'Nothing you don't know about, anyhow,' I tell him, laughing.

'No,' he answers, 'it's helpful.'

The nurse today is Julie again, her back better, and she herself in good spirits because she's making a career move. We talk a bit about mastectomy. 'I had a woman once,' she says, ' who went and got a great whacking tattoo over the area once it was all healed. That was breeelliant,' she laughs in her rolling, Scottish accent. I think I manage an 'oh'.

The headache begins as Anthony drives me home from Mount Vernon that afternoon. My daughters are, under our custody arrangements, with their father for this Rosh Hashana, which is adding to my feeling of depression.

But in the event Rosh Hashanah passes in the muted post-chemotherapy haze, so thick it is barely penetrated even by the shofar, the ram's horn, which, in Israel, can be heard from one side of Jerusalem to the other. These Rosh Hashanah prayers and tunes are very familiar to me, etched in my consciousness as far back as I can remember. I have made many decisions on Rosh Hashanah, not least divorce. Much of the language is about looking ahead to the year to come, and what it will bring. The breast cancer is still new enough that I think how strange it is that of all the possibilities I might have contemplated this time last year, cancer is the one that never even crossed my mind.

A woman my age comes over to talk to me during the synagogue service. I don't know her, but she tells me she has children at Nina's school. She has just finished all her chemotherapy, she tells me, and she says, 'Look, I've come through, my hair's grown back.'

By the time the two-day festival is over, the symptoms have really kicked in. One night I sit at the kitchen table, sleepless, writing the following lines over and over. I find them on our cool, dark-green, slate kitchen counter when I come down the next morning, and I don't even remember writing them.

'Sometimes just so bleak, thinking this is me, lying here, may not sleep tonight, ill, going to lose my breast, hair gone, feeling sick. This is so unreal. Sense of unreality, 'cos of wooziness and just getting through days, going from sleepless night to sleepless night.'

Because this is the end of the first stage of my treatment, I see Glenda Kaplan for a mammogram and scan, to find out what effect the treatments have had. Peter Ostler has been looking disconsolate – his tape measure hasn't shown much reduction in the lump size.

Dr Kaplan looks visibly happier when the higher-tech scan shows the lump has shrunk considerably. 'It's just over three centimetres now,' she says, and she is clearly pleased.

'Oh,' I say, 'because Peter Ostler didn't think it had shrunk much.'

'I know,' she says. It's the first time I've seen her since I was first diagnosed and had the blitz of biopsies, and it feels like a small lifetime, but my 'team' meet each week to discuss the progress of the patients in their care. I'm struck by their genuine reactions: both Dr Kaplan's pleasure at the good measurement, and Dr Ostler's wistfulness at the bad.

Anthony and I also see Mr Al-Dubaisi. He looks solemn when I tell him that I have found out that my mother's mother died of breast cancer. He says he will send me for gene testing further down the line, when my treatment is finished. 'It has insurance implications,' he says, 'implications for your family.' I realize by the coldness I suddenly feel that he's talking about my girls.

We talk round and round the question of whether to have more chemotherapy before the surgery. 'I anticipated these questions,' he says, sitting back in his classic pose, fingertips poised together on the desk before him. The original plan was for four rounds of chemotherapy – the Adriamycin and Cyclophosphamide – followed by a mastectomy, to be topped by four further rounds of the newer, more expensive chemotherapy drug Taxotere. Mr Al-Dubaisi says that although the tumour has shrunk considerably its size compared to my breast is still too big to consider a lumpectomy. 'There wouldn't be any breast left to speak of,' he explains.

Oh. Great.

Should I have more chemotherapy, then, before the operation in an attempt to shrink the lump further, and thereby make a mastectomy unnecessary? Mr Al-Dubaisi considers that. 'Not everybody responds to chemotherapy,' he says, in that way doctors have of not telling you the important stuff until after the event. 'But Dina has done.' Having more chemotherapy is 'certainly not contra-indicated'.

'Here's what I will say,' he continues. 'If the lump shrinks to the point where I can no longer feel it, then I will do a lumpectomy, instead of a mastectomy.' Mr Al-Dubaisi adds that the scan shows the lymph node under my arm has disappeared with the chemotherapy. He also says there is always a greater risk of the cancer returning if you don't do a mastectomy.

Part of me just wants to get this operation over with. But the other part thinks about the unimaginable reality of losing a breast and feeling I can't cope with that; I like my body just the way it is, I never envisaged it being mutilated in any way.

Really, I say to myself, the only thing between me and more chemotherapy is that I'm part of the TAC trial, comparing the effects of the two different types of chemo drug and their use pre- and post-operations. If I have more chemo before the operation I will have to come out of the trial.

Anthony is deeply concerned about the trial, and keeps trying to elicit from Mr Al-Dubaisi what is the point of chemotherapy after mastectomy? 'Surely,' he keeps saying, 'the reason for chemotherapy is to destroy the cancer? The mastectomy removes the tumour, so what reason is there to have chemotherapy after surgery?'

Somehow, we never get a clear answer to this, the discussion getting lost between Anthony's probing and Mr Al-Dubaisi's often opaque English. 'But,' he says, 'I like debating with you, Anthony. My father was a lawyer, it reminds me of talking with him.' Mr Al-Dubaisi, I often think, doesn't use language as his primary means of communication. For himself, he takes in the information he needs through his fingertips, the instruments of his surgery, and when he asks questions he isn't really listening to the answers so much as watching to see what the face, the body, reveals.

We have a three-week break, either to recover from the last chemo before the operation, or before resuming further chemotherapy. Three weeks to choose.

8. Now, Which Side Was it Again?

In the beginning, I used to feel my breasts all the time. I'd meet a friend and say, 'I have breast cancer.' Automatically, my left hand would go to my right breast. I'm going to lose this, I'd say out loud, trying to prepare. But they've been through four babies, these breasts, they've been plumper than apple pie, they've drooped flatter than a bad joke; nothing I told myself could make their destruction tangible.

Now, with three months and four chemotherapy treatments behind me, what amazes me is how little I touch them. Here I am, on a couch once again, behind a curtain, chest bare. It's routine. I lie down, and a strange man feels my breasts – which register no sensation. They have become desensitized – a prelude to what's ahead.

And all conducted with such propriety. Mr. Al-Dubaisi says, 'I need to examine you,' and that is the signal for Sister Briodie, the breast-care nurse with her lilting Irish voice, to pull the drapes, leaving the surgeon and my husband where they are, one either side of the desk. Like a handmaiden, Sister Briodie helps me disrobe.

I never see how she indicates to Mr Al-Dubaisi to join us,

but he doesn't once come in until my top is off and I am lying flat on the couch, as if it is the act of getting undressed which is most private of all. He lays his hands flat, feeling his way along the breasts almost as a blind man might, his fingers giving him information his eyes might miss, while a gentle Irishwoman looks on.

A hundred thoughts circle. I'm really stressed, I hear myself thinking. I need to do some yoga. So happy Elon's settled so brilliantly into kindergarten. Realize how unhappy Nina was in her reception year – that miserable teacher. These sentences run on a loop, while automatically I do what Mr Al-Dubaisi asks: 'Lift your arms, please; press your hands into your waist.'

This is the final consultation before the mastectomy. Mr Al-Dubaisi is pleased. He can't feel the lymph node any more, and the lump has shrunk. He retires from the curtained chamber, and Sister Briodie hands me my clothes, not something anybody has ever done for me as an adult.

Back at the desk, I remember to ask to see a photo of what the scar will look like, again one of the things they recommend you do on websites. Only there isn't a photograph available, but Mr Al-Dubaisi tells me it will be flat, the scar going laterally across. He says he'll use the same scar to reach under the arm, to the lymph nodes, and he draws lines in the air.

I've had two weeks to think this over: to decide whether to proceed with the mastectomy, or have further chemotherapy instead. During the fortnight, the Sukkot festival, we all went to Israel, to where Anthony's oldest son is planning to move. We saw my parents, my first meeting with them in seven years, their first time meeting Elon. They said things like, 'nobody is more concerned than we are' and 'it doesn't seem fair to ask you to make the decision about whether to have more chemotherapy before the surgery', shaking puzzled heads.

But in the end, there wasn't a great decision-making process. It was easy.

I didn't want to leave the trial; I want this illness to have some point, and contributing, in however tiny a way, to research seems to give it some reason. And more, if I put the breast-removing surgery off any longer, I doubt I can face it at all.

'How long will I need to be in hospital?' I ask.

'Ten days,' Mr Al-Dubaisi says.

'A week,' I counter. We are old sparring partners now.

The operation will be tomorrow, at four-thirty, a Friday afternoon. My three daughters will be at their father's. Anthony and I have talked, of course, about rearranging the contact in the best way possible given the circumstances, but we can't work out what that is, so in the end we decide, as we usually do, just to let the die fall as it may. Anthony's children will be with us this weekend, so Elon won't be without siblings at home.

I have to have a blood test before the operation. I hate blood tests. I cry. As we leave Mr Al-Dubaisi, I rattle off a list of errands at Anthony, stuff that must be done this minute, nine, ten random things, paint samples (unbelievably, yet again, we seem to have spawned builders in the house), pants for a newly potty-trained Elon, milk, bread, broad beans.

I finish writing an interview with Meg Cabot, author of

The Princess Diaries. She's been a splash of colour across this week, coming to my house to be interviewed, sporting pink cowboy boots for which she scoured the Internet, she tells me, a purple streak in her glossy black hair, and a silver belt with a crown for a clasp. She walks in bearing flowers: 'I hear you're having a hard time,' she says softly.

Cabot is one of the elite band of children's authors whose books sell on both sides of the Atlantic. Piles of review copies of books arrive in our house most days, and many end up languishing in cardboard boxes waiting to be taken to one of the local schools or hospitals. Cabot's books barely make it out of the envelope before the girls race to snatch them.

She is a pink descendant of Enid Blyton – boiled down, her stories are vintage girls' school tales, about the unpopular kid who gets her own back, suitably aided by serious wealth. It's a theme that resurfaces endlessly on the Disney television channel, and in countless high-school-themed films; the fairy tale of our times. Our teenage girls seem much more clued up than I was as a schoolgirl – their dress sense honed, their wit ready to bat away put-downs – and I put some of it down to how much Cabot-style material they read.

Cabot's narratives draw on her days as a kind of matron in a girls' dormitory at New York University – 'snobbiest school ever', she calls it grimly, detailing the girls' deeply unpleasant behaviour to each other. 'When I was starting out,' Cabot tells me, 'I wanted to be a "serious" writer – you know, write about death, and be taken seriously.' But then she looked back into her own diaries, plundered the material and when she read stuff out, her friends said, that's great. 'I was such a horrible child,' she chuckles. 'My diaries are full of stuff like "I hate my mother" and all my concerns are so self-centred; you know, "I have the hugest spot on my face" and then the next sentence'd be, "Grandma's in hospital."'

This evening, there is squabbling downstairs in our home. Theo and Nina, a year apart, are in full spate. 'You dropped them, you pick them up.' 'No, you . . .'

And then: 'Mu-u-u-u-mmmm!'

Ragged from this illness, Anthony and I break our cardinal rule, and each side with our own child. Alarmed, Nina and Theo take to the couch, while we turn on one another. And so it goes, on into the night before the mastectomy.

Friday morning. This afternoon, I'm heading into hospital for up to ten nights. Sister Briodie mentioned, almost in passing, that I will need front-opening pyjamas. After the operation it will be hard to manage clothes that need pulling over my head.

It's not just the big questions doctors don't answer: will I live, will the lump come back? There's the small stuff too – so paltry nobody addresses it, least of all breast-cancer consultants. Like, what in hell do you wear when they take away one of your breasts?

I don't have a ten-day-in-hospital wardrobe. I don't even maintain an overnight-in-hospital outfit. In fact, I don't run to so much as a dressing gown. So I'm chasing round Brent Cross, a five-minute drive from my house. Brent Cross was London's first shopping mall, and I can remember when it opened, although at the time – I was eight – it didn't seem as remarkable as it does now that the powers that be chose Hendon for this auspicious first.

I am looking for front-opening pyjamas, then for front-opening anything. All the pyjamas are like the ones I own already – T-shirt/sweatshirt tops. The front-opening night-dresses are maternity provender in Mothercare, and I'm starting to think that's what I'll be packing for the mas-tectomy.

Averting my eyes from bras, I brush past something soft in Marks and Spencer's: silk pyjamas in sludgy colours, grey-green and soft rose, the trousers easy pull-ons with forgiving elasticated waists, the tops button-down shirts. In a flamboyant, going-to-hospital flourish, I take two pairs of each.

Tonight is Shabbat, the Jewish Sabbath. The children finish school early and, as it happens, all appear at once, about 3 p.m. – even Max and Laura, Anthony's eldest two, who don't go to school any more. It's a coincidence, the two big ones, as we tend to call them, appearing right now; their rhythms are different, separated off from the day-to-day life of our household, and I'm not sure they know I'm heading off to have an operation. I register Laura's white, tense face, and her confusion at the unusual activity in our front hallway as I pack up to go. Later, days later, I find out she'd just broken up with a boyfriend. There is a Pandora's box aspect to what are called blended families, where every time the front door opens different bits of family history collide.

My daughters bring a hospital-survival box, packed with card-tricks, tiny lavender toiletries and a hand-stitched book Sara-Jenny has put together of family photos and captions they've written. Anthony hands over Sidney Blumenthal's book on the Clintons – pocket *West Wing*. I also take a picture Elon has drawn, titled 'Mummy, I Love You', photos from our trip to Israel, and some prints we've had done of the children. The downside of private health care is you miss out on the ward camaraderie, but this is the upside; you get to make your room your own.

We drive round the corner to the Garden Hospital. Yesterday, I had the phone call saying the operation would be at five-thirty; today, I phone to ask when I need to turn up, and the secretary says, vaguely, 'Oh, about four o'clock, I guess.'

The nurse has props. 'Ha, ha, these are really sexy,' she chuckles, unfurling a pair of immensely heavy, tightly woven stockings. We inch these up and along my legs – super-elastic structures to stop blood clots forming. With a gaping hospital gown, my two stiff, white legs stretched straight out in front of me and my top half flopped on two huge hospital pillows, I look like a giant marionette.

Then the anaesthetist appears, settling down in an armchair to run through his repertoire. 'Any tooth crowns, ha, ha!' he chortles. 'Ah, well, any piercings I can't see, tee hee!' I can choose how to launch the anaesthesia – insert a suppository myself, or have someone help. I say I'll do it, and spend the next forty-five minutes absolutely sure that it's slipped out and won't do the trick.

Mr Al-Dubaisi reads a document of consent to me. 'Your husband, the lawyer, will tell you we have to do this,' he says, his gentle attempt at a joke, but he's upset for me, his voice is unsteady. 'The purpose of treatment is removal, and staging,' he reads out. Staging? 'Yes, we send the tumour off to find out what is in it.'

He asks me to sign and I do, trying to decide what surname I use for operations – married, or single. Turns out it's single. Mr Al-Dubaisi makes a felt-tip cross over my right breast. 'Now, which side is it, again?' he says, the requisite gag.

The nurse reappears to walk us down to the theatre, all very casual, no being portered down on trolleys. From the Gambia, she easily puts her arms round me, and doesn't seem to feel the need to crack any jokes at all. 'You must be strong for her,' she says to Anthony, because we are both crying now.

Anthony's going home to make Friday-night dinner for Max, Laura, Chloë, Theo and Elon. Myrna, Anthony's mum, is there too. I'm anxious for him to get back to the children, to make Friday night normal. He leaves at the door to the operating theatre, and I stroll on in.

More jokes, as they usher me on to the bed. 'It's freezing,' I say.

'Yup, we're the Eskimo brigade in here.'

Then another round of the 'which side are we doing again?' joshing, and 'do you feel woozy yet?'

'No, I really don't.'

'Should we get the good stuff out for her? OK, then.'

∾

'Was supper OK? Was Elon all right? I've asked you already, haven't I?'

'Only nine hundred times,' Anthony says, holding my

hand. 'It was all fine, everybody sends their love, Elon is great, he's gone to sleep.'

I remember having that snatch of conversation, I remember the lights were on in the bedroom, and I thought that was strange because it was Shabbat, and we don't leave the lights on in our bedroom, and I remember Anthony saying to me, 'You won't remember any of this in the morning.'

Then there was a night of deep sleep between wakings, nurses coming in and doing things, helping me to the bathroom.

Next morning, Anthony arrives and tells me all sorts of conversations I don't remember having had at all: that I was in pain and so he called for pethidine, and that he read me the captions on the photos in the booklet the children made, spangled with green and silver stars and labelled, 'strictly unedited'.

In the afternoon everybody turns up at once; my girls walking over from their father, and Anthony back with the rest of the children. I hear them before they come in, my window is open to the road. Inside, they drape themselves round the room, perched on windowsills playing cards, on the edge of the bed looking at photo albums, curled in the one armchair, deep into *Marie-Claire* magazine. Mr Al-Dubaisi comes in, looks at the card game and offers to teach them one that involves gambling.

He wants to check his handiwork, but says he'll come back when everybody is gone.

'It's fine,' I say. 'I'd prefer them to see, than wonder about it.'

I haven't looked at myself yet. Mr Al-Dubaisi, not as

into full exposure as I am, stands foursquare in front of me, shielding the site of the operation from the eight non-medical people in the room, takes a lightning-quick peek, and announces, 'I am satisfied, all is well.'

I have bandages strapped across my right side, and there are two plastic tubes running from beneath the bandages into two pint-sized plastic bottles. Both bottles are filling up with a brownish-red fluid. I have put the bottles into a gold gift bag, very Meg Cabot, so that when I walk, I just lift the handle of the bag. The carrying bag is another tip from the children – in one of the American teen movies they watch incessantly, the heroine does the same in a hospital scene. Before the operation I had read *Topsy and Tim Go to Hospital* several times to Elon, so he'd have some sense of where I was off to, and when I told the older kids that after the mastectomy I'd have these tubes and bottles, they knew all about it: 'Oh sure, you just take in really cool shopping bags.'

Everybody leaves at nightfall. Later, Anthony comes back and we both fall asleep on the bed watching TV.

I make it to the bathroom myself about three o'clock Sunday morning. Sitting on the toilet reading *Marie-Claire*, I realize what it was the girls were looking at so intently earlier this afternoon. I feel a knot clenching in my stomach reading about Caron Keating dying of breast cancer. There are pages of photographs of post-mastectomy women, pages I rush past.

I am desperate for a bath. The wound is leaking, so I have bloodstains on the new silk pyjamas. Again and again I bless them, though, the way they slide on, so cool, so soft, the dull, expensive sheen on them. And,

prosaically, the fact that they are machine-washable. I've already changed three times, blood, sweat and silk all mingling, so I will send them home to be washed.

There is screaming outside in the corridor. The woman across the hall is calling, 'Help! Help!' in a high voice. I stand outside her door, uncertain. The nurse appears, and says the woman – who has Alzheimer's – has a carer all the time in with her, that there is nothing anybody can do to ease her distress.

I can't raise my right arm. I feel invalided. I am without full movement. This is why the pyjamas need to be front-buttoning. To change, I sit on the bed, with the bottles in the bag next to me, slip an arm out of one side, and then the other. I cannot raise my arm even as high as my shoulder. I did not expect this.

When morning light finally filters through the curtains, the nurse who walked me down to the operating theatre comes in and gives me a kiss on both cheeks. 'I know when I see you, you're one of my good ones,' she says. 'It's no good saying you can't fight it; you have to say, my little boy needs me, and I'm here for him.'

Eleven o'clock Sunday morning. I inspect the dressing on my breast – ex-breast? – in the mirror for the first time. Lying propped on hospital pillows, looking down at myself, my body doesn't seem that different. But in the mirror, stark as a minus sign, I'm faced with a full sense of the new flatness.

Grief is waiting to swamp me. To ward it off, I take snapshots of myself on my phone, and realize glasses and bald head is not a good look. I'll put my lenses in; the bottles draining from my chest balanced on the sink, my newly immobile right arm clutched to my side, as I manoeuvre contact-lens solutions with my left hand.

I talk to the nurses. There are African princesses working in this hospital, daughters of Gambian tribal chiefs, others from Sierra Leone, a country ruined by diamonds, they say. They come over here to make money; their children back home are aged fourteen and twenty-one. The money sends the fourteen-year-old to school. Their families think life here is very comfortable. They don't know how expensive accommodation is, how every saved penny goes back to Africa, that there is no luxury here. And now, they don't fit in anywhere any more, they don't fit in here, and they don't fit in there.

A client of Anthony's has sent a giant confection of deep-red orchid. It took two guys to bring it upstairs to my room. All the African nurses go mad for it, stroking its leaves.

Finally an Australian physiotherapist comes in and says that, as far she is concerned, 'You're ready to go home.' She calls this lead-heavy hauling up of my arm 'full movement'. I stare at her, dumb at her blithe 'your range of movement's excellent; here is a leaflet of exercises'.

Anthony arrives with Elon, and flops, exhausted, into a chair. He says it's strange how he feels so brittle, so fragile, and I'm the one who's had surgery. I barely hear him; I'm scared of Elon pulling the two tubes that now run from my chest, so every empathetic skill I possess is focusing on this three-year-old energy force firmly straddling the hospital bed. I show Elon the tubes as soon as I see him looking at them. 'Hmmm, what's this?'

Look, reddish liquid going from Mummy's bandages

into two glass bottles. Allowed to touch them, he loses interest – the oldest trick. Next up, the magic cupboard next to my bed, just for Elon, which today opens to disclose five little knights on horses. So far, I've forgotten to give the older children the bits and bobs from Clare's Accessories I bought for them.

By night-time, I want my dressing changed, I want my sheets changed, I want these heavy bottles changed, and I still want a bath. There is no hot water in my room, and there will be no clean sheets until tomorrow apparently. The nurses are kind – they shake their heads over the stained state of my bedding, but tell me they're sorry, there is no fresh laundry over the weekend. Also, new bottles will have to wait for a delivery from Queen Charlotte's, their sister hospital.

I ask, 'Please, can you change these bandages?' This afternoon Mr Al-Dubaisi came again – younger-looking in his weekend clothes, soft camel jacket instead of the suit and tie – and I heard him tell the nurse to change the dressing, after I complained it was leaking.

'Oh,' she says, 'he came back to me after, and said I should wait until tomorrow.' But she can see how it's soaked through, new red blood making rivulets along the dried brown patches, and she makes a wry, conspiratorial face: 'What do doctors know?'

Out comes a sheath of crisp, paper-wrapped dressings, and with what feels like an anciently learned slowness, she unpeels the tape on my chest, watching my face the whole time. All I feel is some tugging. They may not run hot water in my room, but the painkillers are on tap, two little red ones and a longish white one, every few hours.

In the earliest hours, the Alzheimer's patient across the hall wakes: 'You can't keep me here,' she yells.

I look in the full-length mirror again. Fluent breast-feeder, I could always summon milk at will. And what do you know? I can still do it. I am absolutely sure of the sensation, that old internal rush, and I can feel it to my right breast, site of Friday's mastectomy, just like when I needed milk to come to feed my babies. I'm standing in front of a full-length mirror, watching myself tentatively, so tentatively, touch my way all around the soft, new, white bandages, and the tears are running down my face because I've made a mistake and let the grief in after all.

9. 'It's for Your Hair, Mummy'

Mr Al-Dubaisi reports back. Mastectomy, he says, yet again, was the right decision. 'There was DCIS – pre-cancer – in every quartile of the breast.' This didn't show up in the mammograms. Also, he removed *thirteen* lymph nodes, he says with some emphasis. It is a justification of the surgeon's manual skills in this high-tech age: the information we had prior to the operation – that there was one lymph node which had disappeared with chemotherapy – was simply what the machines revealed.

Meanwhile, each day Elon creates more of a fuss about leaving me behind in hospital. And I'm just getting into the swing of it: three meals a day delivered to my bed on a tray, the remote-controlled television all to myself.

Today, Elon lopes in behind a gigantic purple card, hand-made with his teacher Alison, whose sister is just finishing her breast-cancer treatment. Not for the first time, this illness feels like a necklace of women across the world.

The card is a froth of glitter and highly scrumpled clumps of tissue paper, and says, 'To Mummy, lots and lots of kisses, hugs and I hope you get better soon. I love you, love Elon xxx.' A note at the bottom in the same thick black felt-tip reads, 'Dictated by Elon'. 'It's for your hair, Mummy,' he says as he climbs on the hospital bed to give it to me.

I wear a bandanna for the school run (I never did wear that £1300 wig – it went into a high-up cupboard, on its own, on a stand, to scare the wits out of anybody who should venture there) but at home, and now in hospital, I am bareheaded. I worried Elon might find this frightening, but he has only ever found it ticklish, his face to my scalp. I realize now though, from his card, something I didn't take in before – that in his mind he has understood breast cancer as an illness that makes your hair unwell.

Actually, understanding this cancer has taken me a while. These hospital days feel like the first time I've stopped to think.

Like how I felt demeaned by a wig – it was a denial. For myself, for my three daughters, in this ultra body-conscious age, I don't want to hide this newly commonplace passage of womanhood, but rather wear it like Demi Moore did her pregnancy on the cover of *Vanity Fair*. Back home after this operation I will still walk around my bathroom without clothes on, and I know the smaller children will still wander in.

There's such a thing as too much exposure, though, even for me. This Monday morning in hospital, fresh sheets arrive, and an East European nurse appears, complete with student, to take me to my first bath since the surgery.

In the tub, she washes my back and, not for the first time, I think: the kindness of nurses.

But also, the indignity of it. Climbing into a bath with two people watching. Stripped of hair. Tubes attached. Carrying two bottles of fluid around in a Starbucks bag now.

The nurse asks if I want to be left alone, and I say, 'Yes, please.' She shows me how the taps work, but seconds later I realize I haven't paid attention. And I have to quash my panic because the hot water is running and I don't know how to turn it off, and I can't climb out of the bath fast because I can't use one arm. 'Calm down,' I tell myself, 'and breathe deeply.'

One-armed, I hoist myself out and concentrate on working out how to adjust the water. The taps are a lever system – designed for the injured, I guess, but too complicated for me, like childproof medicine bottles that only defeat grown-ups.

'Just breathe . . . breathe deeply,' I coach myself. It's my first, acute sense of being invalided. Again, nobody prepared me for this or, maybe, they glossed over it and I wasn't listening carefully enough.

I love baths; love the feel of being surrounded and supported by warm water. I had my third and fourth labours in water pools – like giant Jacuzzis deep enough to cover you in water standing should you feel like it. But I wasn't able to deliver the babies underwater, because as soon as I sank into the bath, the labour pains ceased. 'If you ever want this baby to come out, Dina,' the midwife said at last, 'you're going to have to step out of the water.'

When my hair first came out I wasn't sure what to use on my scalp, didn't know if I was supposed to keep on shampooing or what, really. Our bath at home is edged with squat white bottles of balneum oil, which is what I always use on the children to prevent them from suffering the eczema I had as child. Because shampoo felt too harsh for my newly denuded scalp I used to rub balneum in, then rinse it all with warm water. In the early days of hair loss my scalp felt tender all the time. I would just lie back in the oil-slicked water and soak my scalp.

This hospital morning having a bath, as always, makes me feel better. I step out, crouching on knees first of all, then use one arm to hoist myself to standing. I climb over the edge and grimace because the towels are handkerchief-sized. I dab my wet skin, one-handed, my bruised body looming too large against this fluttering scrap of hospital towelling.

On Wednesday morning the nurses take the appallingly named 'drains' out, the plastic tubing carrying blood and something rust-coloured from my mastectomy wound to the plastic bottles etched with markings to measure their contents. They give me painkillers half an hour before to numb the area, but it's still excruciating, that killer mix of whatever the actual sensation is combined with my fear of how it will feel, topped off by the look on the nurse's face that says, sorry, this hurts. I'm left with a bruised right side and a fleshy fold of skin. I'm going home; I've been here five nights.

Nobody has offered me a prosthesis – the name, apparently, for whatever it is you're supposed to wear when your breast has been removed. How does it stay on, I wonder? Velcro? A band of elastic around your back? In Mr Al-Dubaisi's other parish, his NHS hospital, Barnet General, a breast-care nurse would visit, but I have chosen this small, private unit, because it is in my neighbourhood, a place my children pass on their way to school, and there is no assigned breast cancer nurse here.

This is an illness that has not quite shaken off its taboos. Death is not the secret any more, but what the treatment does to women – attacking the hair, the breasts, turning the mother of the species into a pre-pubescent boy.

I try on vest tops. Bent forward from the waist, I can slither them on, but break into a sweat trying to twist them off again. That movement I have never in my life even thought about – the one you do to take a T-shirt over your head – is near-impossible now, a consequence of the lymph-node surgery under my arm. I slink back into the silk pyjamas and put a jacket over them.

The physiotherapist hasn't told me how long it will take my arm to heal – just that I can't drive for some weeks, or pick up heavy loads, or push a buggy. How's that supposed to work, I wonder? I also know reconstruction will wait for at least two years – radiotherapy can affect the cosmetic surgery. But these thinking days I feel it is wise too – immediate reconstruction seems, mentally, too great a leap to take: a suppression, another denial. And, as it happens, I don't think a prosthesis – whatever one looks like – is me either.

The nurse here seems to sense that I am flailing somewhat, and asks if I want to speak to one of the staff who had a mastectomy last year. So this pleasant woman comes into my room and asks if I have any questions. But I can't think what to ask.

These are the questions: What do I wear when I can

only put on clothes that are front-opening, but not stiff shirts because that will hurt my currently bruised and raw flesh? How do I shop, cook, feed, bath a child, lift a child for cuddles and when requested when every instinct is to keep my battered right arm tight against my side, nursing the savaged part against myself, scared to lift the elbow out at all in case my body tears – which is what it feels like it will do. How do I keep my column deadline when the advice I've been given is 'no repetitive actions, such as typing' because of the fear of something called lymphoedema?

Anthony comes to pick me up. I've packed up my room, the photos, the pictures Elon did, the cards that came with flowers, the dried fruit in bowls, my toiletries and the jewellery I chose so carefully for my stay, the shining things I thought I should take with me to keep my individuality intact.

I didn't wear any jewellery in hospital. The first thing that happens is you have to take off everything metallic before they begin operating, and afterwards I was too bruised, too swollen, to want anything touching any part of my body. What I needed, but didn't have, was more clothing: many more pairs of underpants, and many more pairs of pyjamas, made of material to caress the skin, because all the clothes soaked through with sweat and blood.

Leaving the hospital room this Wednesday lunchtime I don't put a bandanna on, realizing with a jolt that I won't be able to, because I can't tie one on without the use of both arms. I have a green jacket from Prada, at least eight years old, and it slips on over the silk pyjamas, and I walk out with Anthony, saying goodbye to the nurses. In the lift there's that sense of how this should be an occasion somehow, marked with processions of elephants, perhaps, only it isn't.

Down in the lift, and heading out the front door. 'Just one moment, Mrs Julius,' a woman calls from behind the reception desk. I turn to hear good wishes for my recovery, or just goodbye, really. 'Can I get you to sign this, please?' It's a bill for £14.23, drinks that Anthony had and some telephone calls, which are not covered by the insurance apparently. The bill for the rest of this stay is in the thousands . . .

We walk to the car park. There's that eerie sense of re-entering the world, not having been through a door to the outside for days, of shedding a protective layer. Next week Anthony must be in court, and so, driving or not, I am doing the school run. And the question is, what do you wear when you're left with one breast?

At home, I'm in the silk pyjamas still, wearing the top next to my skin, and putting cardigans on over that. I bath Elon from the first night, doing the forbidden lifting, using it as a stomach-pulling-in exercise. I lift him with my left arm, and every muscle my stomach possesses.

My parents phone. 'Which children are in the house?' they ask. This is a question only ever asked of those of us who have divorced and whose children continue to see the other parent. 'Which children are in the house?' Not even, which children are home – because for my parents' generation we are not making homes, we are the generation of 'Mummy's house' and 'Daddy's house'. They created homes; we accumulate houses.

Home is lying in my bed this one morning with tea and strawberries and looking out at the leaves just changing colour. It's also avoiding the phone, feeling wildly grateful that Anthony's taken Elon out this afternoon, and equally resentful that I just got home from hospital and I'm making supper! But Anthony keeps Elon out all afternoon, so at least I'm making supper in peace. I make mushroom soup, my fall-back comfort food: mushrooms, onion, garlic, leek, all in the pot cooking in some olive oil, then water and, if you have them, you can add some nutmeg, strong squeezes of lime or lemon, and white wine. I use lots of wine, and cream or milk at the end. Other days I make vegetable soup: carrots, onion, celeriac, swede, butternut squash, parsnips, all chopped up. Repetitive arm motions. It is not possible to chop vegetables with my left hand.

I'm also answering emails. The South Bank Show is planning a programme on Jacqueline Wilson; can they talk to me? Of course. I can't raise my arm, but I can talk. I drive to Hampstead – driving, another forbidden action – to meet the two producers: Lucy Allen, the film-maker, is also a jewellery designer, and she's wearing one of her own necklaces, dozens of brightly flamboyant beads knotted several times around her neck, and just looking at the colours is enough to make mastectomy a thing of the past. Over the next months I will buy some of Lucy's necklaces, and wear them like talismen, and when I hit bad patches she sends me one she's made specially, burnt reds and golds.

We talk about Wilson's jewellery, of course, her trademark rings, several of them on each finger, a tactic for triggering conversations with children. But we also talk about mothers. Jacqueline Wilson's relationship with her mother is an unresolved one, I think, and it's the source of a lot of her stories. They tell me Melvyn Bragg, the show's anchor, cares hugely about his mother's opinion of him. Bragg's two South Bank producers and I all share a wry smile at this, and at how very long the shadows are that mothers cast. The whole business of mothering is fraught, our expressions say.

It's been the theme underlying all our chatting this pre-filming morning. Holding down jobs in a very competitive business, these two young women producers are at the point of deciding whether they can ever be mothers, or whether it will ruin their hard-fought-for careers. It is recuperative, this moving from hospital days back into a world where people weigh job satisfaction against motherhood.

I've interviewed Jacqueline Wilson twice. Wilson is the most-borrowed author from British libraries; this year, for the first time, I noticed mothers in the playground reading her titles. Her books come out now in the brightest of jackets, cerulean blues and vermilion pinks. Wilson's image is honed; her hands studded with giant and intricate silver rings. When she was a child, she told me, her mother always put her in velour coats, little hats and absolutely no jewellery.

The first time we met, in 2001, was just as her reputation was becoming really huge, I guess. We met in the Piccadilly branch of Waterstone's, a favourite haunt of hers, on a road of her favourite places, Fortnum and Mason, and Hatchards, the bookshop. The children's department, right by a juice bar, was deserted that school morning, but the stands were piled high with Wilson's books.

She came to the interview with a woman friend. After Wilson separated from her husband she started going on London walks, the kind advertised in the London listings magazine *Time Out*, where a group meets at a designated point and a guide points out sights you wouldn't notice otherwise. On one of these walks, Wilson met the American lady who was with her that first morning we met.

These days – she is now children's laureate, and has eight-hour queues whenever she does a book signing – there can't be many people who don't at least recognize Jacqueline Wilson's name, although when she and I meet again, some weeks after I start writing 'The Enemy Within', she chuckles good-naturedly about a garden party the Queen gave to which some of the children's writers were invited.

'She spoke to all of us,' Wilson told me. 'She came over and said to me, "And what do you do?" So I said, "I write children's books," and I could see the royal countenance glazing over, so I said, "But your grandchildren are probably too old for my stuff now." "Ah, but we have another one coming along," she said, pointing to Sophie Wessex. I thought that was pretty quick on the feet of her!'

Wilson, the kind of person who pays attention to others, remembered that I live in a house with many children. We'd been talking about her marriage, and how – she recalled with no little bemusement in her voice and on her face – she'd laundered and ironed her ex-husband's shirts for years as a matter of course. 'It was a three-shirt-a-day job: work shirt, leisure shirt, formal shirt,' she tells me. She had no domestic help in the house, 'partly because I'm a control freak', she said, and 'partly because I'd be embarrassed. Anyhow, neither of us gave a damn about the house – we had to lie down and rest at the thought of hammering a nail. And I'm not house-proud. I generally fall into a heap at the thought of doing house-work. I think I was a good, interested mother,' she added, 'but I didn't do little meals on the table, it was a case of opening a tin and hoping for the best.'

I said my big thing was supper, having enough food in the house and then preparing it. Not to mention the clearing away in readiness for the next morning's packed lunches. 'But how do you do that?' she asked me with genuine wonder. 'I know,' I said. 'I'm amazed how much of my mind it occupies.'

10. The New Amazons

Everything in the house seems to be breaking. The dishwasher is broken, there's a leak in the bathroom – £500 later and a new gasket, and that's sorted – and what was supposed to be a two, maybe three-week job of putting cupboards into Marganit's room has turned into an exercise of pleading with the carpenter just to turn up.

Nothing happens easily, these days. The doctors have made me take out my progesterone-packed contraceptive coil, because they don't want any extra hormones in my body, and I realize I need to have a conversation with them about contraception – is there anything we can use apart from condoms?

Actually, just in case mastectomy isn't effective enough at preventing sexual activity, we do, of course, have an in-house method: Elon is still a trainee sleeper, and regularly wakes up once or twice during the night, not to mention starting most days at around a quarter to six in the morning. In any event, I'm tired, and don't see much of any evening, falling asleep by nine usually, once Elon's in bed and Nina's homework is sorted. Anthony sits up with the older children watching *One Tree Hill*, shepherding others back safely into the house from their teenage lives. On the odd occasion when we have post-mastectomy sex it feels careful, of course, edging round the borders of any operated areas, but it is also momentous, in a way that I remember sex feeling the first time after each child's birth – but this time there's a sadness that sweeps my body. I think it's a recognition of loss.

Never mind, today is going to be fluffy, it will be everything that is not flat, it will be like champagne in roof gardens, Cole Porter on speed. I am to be styled: by *Vogue*. With what feels like a crippled right arm, a bruised right side and scar-skin that is so sensitive it even seems to hiss at the Nivea cream I've been advised to use on it, the only clothes I have been able to wear on my top half are the silk pyjama tops I bought for hospital: I layer one over the other to go outside. So I email the features editor at *Vogue*. I want to write a piece for them, I say, about just how hard it is to get dressed when you're going through chemotherapy and you're reshaped by mastectomy.

They are keen on the idea, and as we discuss it, talk about photographs. I ask whether they have a stylist who can help, who would have some ideas about what clothes might work. 'I'm stuck in pyjamas,' I say. The keepers of the clothing wisdom say they will send me a top gun. 'When Nicole (Kidman) is in town, Fiona styles her,' is how the person they've chosen for the job is described to me.

People who work at *Vogue* are like palace courtiers of old; they speak a smooth tongue designed to keep outsiders at arm's length while facilitating court business as swiftly as possible. So you need to decode their language. But, while the gap between the zero effort required to make Nicole Kidman radiate celebrity and whatever it will take to get me out of my pyjamas is wider than the planet, it does sound like *Vogue* takes the task seriously. This is good, because I am about the lowest I have yet been, the most desperate, fending off even thinking about what I'm going through because I'm afraid of sagging into depression.

My mastectomy wound is swelling bizarrely, inflating and deflating, on and off. I'm petrified of the condition called lymphoedema, a medical state I'd never even heard of three weeks ago, but which now looms menacingly just beyond any of the countless actions I have always carried out with my right arm. Lymphoedema is a swelling of the hand and arm, caused by the removal of the lymph nodes and their lymph-draining activity.

After the usual dithering about whether my symptoms are 'enough' to go and see the doctor, I make an appointment with Mr Al-Dubaisi, just two days after I return home from hospital. He tells me all is well, except he will need to aspirate, which means, he explains when I ask, puncturing the swelling with a needle.

'No, no more needles,' I say.

'You have to trust me, Dina,' Mr Al-Dubaisi says. 'This won't hurt'.

It doesn't; it is as if he has pierced sponge. This is both a relief, and profoundly upsetting. My right breast can now be punched by a needle and I – super-sensitive as I am to long, thin bits of steel penetrating my body – cannot feel a thing.

Sister Briodie, the breast-care nurse, gives me a piece of genuinely good advice: the trick with the physiotherapy exercises, she says, is not how strenuously you do them, but rather doing little and often. Five exercises, each repeated three times, and done five times a day. Such limited movements: raising my arm to touch a wall in front of me, then, from whatever point I manage to reach, crawling up the wall with my fingers, trying to reach a higher spot each day; then turning and attempting the same lift sideways on to the wall, each minute creep upwards a major triumph. I did not imagine this. I was not warned about this.

Sister Briodie's method – each exercise more frequently, but less energetically – stops the peculiar on-off swelling, and this, despite all the forbidden actions I've taken, crippled arm hugged tightly to my side: lifting a hefty three-year-old child, repetitive movements at the keyboard and, of course, driving.

High on Sister Briodie's advice and its quick results, my belief in medical professionals is recharged so fully I even put on the regulation-issue 'cumfie' – the foam-filled flabby pink thing you're supposed to stuff down your bra to approximate the missing breast. The day I go to see Mr Al-Dubaisi about the swelling around the scar, a nurse brings out a plastic bag into which a whole range of these beige artefacts have been thrust, and she says that I can delve in, have a good feel around, and choose whichever I think might be the nearest size.

So that night, Friday night, my first Shabbat at home since the operation, following an afternoon when many people have brought food (the rabbi's wife, Judy Ginsbury, mother of nine, has brought a complete three-course meal for the whole family) I come out of silk pyjamas for the first time since the mastectomy. I have two wrap-around dresses, sub-Diane Furstenburg, very of the moment, very possible for me to put on. I have a soft T-shirt bra from Marks and Spencer's from which, also on the nurse's advice, I have pulled out the underwires. Crying, I reach round to fasten the bra: the tears are because it hurts, and because this is so not a piece of clothing designed for how I look right now.

I feel like a Stepford wife, like Jacqueline Wilson ironing her husband's shirts – like I'm conforming to the world, instead of the world adjusting to me. I pull the cumfie out of its plastic casing. It is flesh-coloured, like the way Crayola wax crayons do flesh, bearing no resemblance to actual skin, and it has sponge stuffing. You can, the nurse showed me, extract wads of the stuffing to make the cumfie match your other breast in size. I wear the dress, and slip on boots. I go downstairs and the children don't comment, but on their faces I see a fleeting relief that I appear quite normal. But it doesn't feel like a relief to me. Once you've recruited an extra arm to get the bra on – and even forgetting the still-fairly-recently-weaned three-year-old putting his hand down your front in public – fastening a bra on this bruised and battered flesh is grimly uncomfortable. This isn't one the medical establishment can answer.

Which is where *Vogue* comes in. They call this the fashionable cancer, the one that attracts big-money charity events and oodles of celebrity endorsement, but nobody's tackling the basic fashion question: what do you wear? Certainly not the skinny breast-cancer awareness T-shirts with round targets on them: T-shirts are out of the question for those who cannot lift their arms, and more-over have only one breast.

This is uncharted territory for *Vogue*'s Fiona Golfar as much as for me, a reluctance that shows on her face as she walks into the café where we've arranged to meet. It's Monday morning, exactly eleven days since I came out of hospital. Working out possible clothes for the post-mastectomy one-in-nine is not, I get the impression, what this fashionista, married to the theatre impresario Robert Fox, thinks of as her beat.

But as she walks in, though her eyes are wary, she's talking, talking before she even sits down: about her Hendon connections, her mother, about reading my 'very practical' columns over the weekend.

She reaches over and touches the collar of the teal silk pyjama top. 'This is nice,' she says, 'where's it from?'

'This is it, the pyjama top I keep going on about – the only clothing I can wear at the moment. From Marks and Spencer's,' I tell her.

'Hmmm,' says the *Vogue* journalist, 'I think we'll try Bond Street.'

They have changing rooms the size of whole cancer units in South Molton Street, a small pedestrianized patch just off the more famous Bond Street, and home to Browns', one of London's longest-established high-fashion shops. The nice, older woman who brings me heaps of clothes to try on tells Fiona she has many women come in post-mastectomy, though I can see from her face when she catches sight of my Nivea-encased scar that she has most certainly never had women come in this soon after the operation.

'Pyjama party . . . at Eleven Downing Street, Gordon and Sarah Brown . . .' Ignoring all shop-assistant gazes, I'm gamely trying to chat during this trial by luxury clothing, but my words are coming out slightly muffled, because I'm gingerly levering my immobile post-mastectomy arm into some wispy Zoran silks, while trying to affect unconcern about thick, white cream smearing itself on these clothes that are as expensive as they are lightweight. But it's still a good line.

Forget thousand-pound-a-ticket charity bashes, the tightest-kept secret of all is that you have to be in children's book reviewing if you want to name-drop the really swell parties. Lucky I am, then, because while *Vogue*'s Fiona has been rattling off A-list gossip all morning, all I've been able to counter with is my 'Hendon theory' – the one that posits that all important news stories have a Hendon connection.

But when Fiona asks me if there's anything particular I need clothes for – other than my date next week with the second, and vastly more expensive phase, of my chemotherapy treatment – I can say: 'Yes, the chancellor of the exchequer and his wife are hosting a launch for a story collection, *Stars at Bedtime*.' The invitations, studded with the names of attending celebrities, came through some months ago now, complete with correctly sized and gendered sets of pyjamas for accompanying children. The pyjamas are from Boden, a newish mail-order company with a nice line in decidedly old-world children's clothing.

Grown-ups, however, are expected to come in day-wear, although so far this shopping trip has yet to persuade me out of my current wardrobe staple, the button-down silk pyjamas. Though these changing rooms are seductively lit, furnished with chaises longues and spacious (and for a moment I'm flooded with the full horror of just how awful it would have been to have undertaken this search for post-mastectomy clothing in Brent Cross, with its communal spaces and fluorescent bulbs) and though these clothes are indeed soft, there is no way they withstand the combination of the chemotherapy-induced menopausal hot sweats, and the cream for the scar. The M&S silk, you see, is washable.

I try on reams of cashmere softer than a baby's breath, and silk lighter than air. 'Listen,' I say to Fiona, 'it is finer fabric, but it doesn't do more for me than what I already have, and the M&S satin pyjamas, which I wear as jackets, you know,' I expand enthusiastically, 'why they go in the machine and if you take them out of the dryer fast enough and hang them up, you don't even have to iron them.'

'OK, OK,' Fiona says, but then, heading out of Brown's, she stops. 'Have you found the Missoni scarves yet?' she asks the assistant. The woman in Brown's has patiently brought me outfits to try and discard all afternoon, and she seemed to understand about softness, and clothes that needed to wrap, but my sense of the shop assistants is that they are used to seeing women who are looking for disguises.

I am now adamant that I don't want clothes that fake it. I want a look that works with the reality of my body. Not the 'cumfie' – soft, foam-filled stuffing for the gap in my bra, because a bra is the archetypal insult added to injury. And no wigs either; a wig pays no homage to the sufferings of my scalp.

The Missoni scarf has multicoloured stripes and fringes. 'Great,' Fiona says as she slips it over my head, wrapping it expertly twice over, and wow, it's a transformation. No longer in pain, struggling into clothes that don't help me, this is a scarf that passes my acid test: namely, something you would wear even if you had hair. Long and narrow, its length allows me to reach along the ends to tie it, even without full movement in my arms. And the long stripes perform another function, draped round the neck and trailing down the front of my body over the soft, not-confining clothes that are comfortable now. This is scar-chic: drawing the eye with colour and flair, not tightness and Lycra.

'And beanies,' Fiona exclaims. She's right; a street style my daughters will approve of, but none of us had considered. As soon as I start slipping these warm tea-cosy-type hats over my denuded scalp I'm already spinning their fashion possibilities in my mind, as if I'm actually sheathing myself in *Vogue*-style indoctrination. So, yes, I'm enthusing to Fiona, beanies are the answer to no-wrap days, to mornings you have to get out fast. Also to my lifestyle, with much bending over toddlers' bottoms, and dishwashers – not the time you want long strands of silk getting in the way.

I buy the softest orange cashmere beanie, a shape that sits perfectly on a head without hair and looks like it's been designed to do just that.

Behind a white door off Marylebone High Street, we deal with the on-off half-growth chemotherapy has made of my eyebrows.

It is a closely kept secret that chemotherapy is fantastic

for the complexion. 'Amazing, translucent, like after giving birth,' the *Vogue* people marvel. But it makes short shrift of the eyebrows, leaving them scared-looking, like little storm-tossed caterpillars.

'It's Vaishaly herself,' Fiona says, as the smallest, friendliest person opens a heavy cream-painted door.

Vaishaly Patel, eyebrow-shaper extraordinaire – Liz Hurley, Elle Macpherson, now me – says, 'I can always find a line,' and proceeds to do just that, revealing along the way that she hails from, where else, Hendon.

Vaishaly, reputedly the sculptress of many a royal eyebrow, doesn't use tweezers on her clients, but a technique called 'threading', which is a lot like having a very small lawn mower applied to your brows. She was, she tells me, taught the technique by her aunts. 'Is that who you get to do yours?' I ask her.

'Oh no,' she shudders, 'I never let them touch mine, they only have one kind of line, the aunties,' and she draws a horrified arc in the air.

'So what do you do?' I ask.

'I tweeze,' she says with a grin. 'I couldn't trust anybody else with my eyebrows.'

And then, Fiona's *coup de théâtre*; an idea wrested from her residual memories of her own – glamorous – maternity months, as our shopping day has lengthened, and we're still no closer to dressing me from the neck down. Pleats Please is Issey Miyake's cheaper range. There are no flat plains to these clothes, just myriads of fine folds.

It's a solution to breast-challenged dressing. These clothes, composed of knife-pleat folds, are a polyester material which is not only washable, it also stretches then regains its shape, so you can open it wide to fit over painfully unmoving limbs, or ease it over bruised and battered chests. And more: the way the pleats work with the body and the light, they create mystery around flatness. These clothes never need ironing; once out of the wash you just twist them and leave them to dry.

On top of this, Fiona layers cashmere, wrap-around lengths of this bright-coloured soft wool that cruise the body's deficiencies, and make the no-breasted feel deeply feminine. On my own I'd have rejected – without trying – the cashmere wraps, designed to cross over the breast, but actually this turns out to be the canniest bit of fashion advice. Wear clothes that go to the breast; scarves that drape the area, bring colour to it, but also add prettiness with their flow. Make a feature of lopsidedness. One of my best buys this winter afternoon is an orange poncho, short and snappy, but crucially designed on a slant, one side longer than the other. I wear the long side so it just falls to where my breast used to sit. This is scar-chic too: an item of clothing that reflects my shape now, but instead of highlighting this in an uncomfortable way, it makes a virtue of the unevenness: it becomes a style statement.

These things work. I look in my cupboard after the days I spend shopping with Fiona and I see colour and comfort and clothes that make even the teenagers in my house look up and say, 'You look great.' It is a cure.

∾

'It's fine, none of the kids will be wearing the Boden pyjamas,' I tell Anthony, before we leave for Downing Street.

'Not dead,' Nina says of the chances of her wearing the charmingly old-fashioned Boden nightdress, while Elon firmly accessorizes his beloved, aged and violently garish Spiderman pyjamas with Thomas the Tank Engine slippers that toot when you press the toes.

Down the utterly traffic-free road the Browns inhabit, and through the front door, where I realize at once that mine are the only children not turned out in pastel clothes devoid of any, er, cultural references.

Gordon Brown, man-in-waiting to the premiership of this island, bears down on Elon: 'Welcome, thank you for coming,' he says.

'Yes, hi, I'm Elon, guess what pyjamas I'm wear–' Elon is in full flow when a puzzled look crosses his face. Accustomed all his life to total adoration, this is his first political encounter. No sooner does the chancellor of the exchequer begin to bend towards Elon than his eye is caught by another arrival, and – not a small man – Mr Brown has just shot across the room faster than a super-hero, to press fervently an altogether higher-up hand, that of Bob Geldof.

Elon, fledgling lobbyist, rapidly pads across the room into the mass of minor television celebrities busy helping their offspring with the laid-on party activities, such as stuffing teddy bear suits with cotton wadding, and very soon manages to summon the attention of every single person in the room with incessant and oft-repeated blasts from his very vocal slippers.

11. Falling

I'm downing zillions of pills. Steroids, in preparation for the deluxe chemotherapy drug Taxotere (£2,298.47 a shot), which is the next stage of treatment, and antibiotics because the scar from the surgery has become infected. I scraped through my biology lessons at school – and that was mostly about rabbits anyhow – but I'm sure the infection has been caused by the Nivea with which I've been dousing the scar, on the recommendation of a top plastic surgeon. After two dogged weeks, I've finally given up on the big blue pot of whipped cream gunk and switched to the much lighter aqueous cream instead, which sinks into the skin, rather than sitting on top of it.

I flaunt my antibiotics at other mothers I see during the day. 'Look what I've got,' I sing-song in the playground, brandishing my Fluoxycillin tablets, as show-offy as the kids with their daily haul of new gimmicks. 'It's sensational, these days they prescribe whatever I ask for.'

It is a recurring joke amongst those of us who brave doctors' surgeries with our children's bouts of illness how impossible it is to get a family doctor to prescribe antibiotics, no matter how dire your child's cough. The way GPs make mothers feel was a factor in why I waited so long before asking a doctor about the growing lump on my breast. I was pregnant when I first noticed the lump, and so it wasn't like I even had to make an appointment to see a doctor – I was having regular antenatal checks. I can remember lying on a bed, being examined, and thinking, 'Should I say something? Is a small bump in my right breast the sort of thing to ask a doctor about? Nah, I'm just going to feel stupid . . .'

Taxotere is given as a drip from a plastic bag hanging from the tall metal pole, automatically dispensing the chemotherapy drop by drop. This is different from my first rounds of chemotherapy, which were manually injected, with Julie or that day's duty nurse standing next to the bed throughout gently squeezing the liquid through the syringe into my vein. The more needles I experience, the less relaxed I become when I see one. But the drip – though it's still attached to a needle in the back of your hand – is easier than the hand-held syringe, because it seems to be a more even process than the manual injection, so I'm not aware of that sensation of fluid crawling up my arm.

Also, though they didn't cover this aspect of human physiology either in biology lessons with Dr Rosmarin at my senior school, I think there's a connection between the speed the drug is injected and the after-effects of the treatment. The one time I had the ward sister, who was rushed, and pushed the trigger much faster than the staff nurses, was the time I felt at my most ill and cranky.

Dr Ostler arrives. Mr Al-Dubaisi would never, ever, not by a flicker of an eye muscle, let the knowledge of my journalism cross his face. Peter Ostler cheerily campaigns, briefing me. So, he talks today about one of his hobbyhorses: getting people to participate in trials, to bring the cure closer. 'It used to take eight years to get enough trial patients,' he says. 'GPs would tell us they didn't have the time or the money to give the extras that running a trial requires. But now there is special funding allocated for trial patients, so we get four thousand patients over two years.'

I'm hopping TV channels, going from home improvement to garden makeover. After some caged-lion pacing, Anthony, who can't bear day-time TV, puts a DVD in the laptop. I think, 'Hey, this is my hospital room, my illness, let me watch what I want.' Television is crucial when you have cancer; getting it absolutely right is important. I made a mistake the first couple of chemo treatments, watching DVDs of my favourite programmes. Now I only have to hear the title music, or see a picture of the stars, and I'm flooded with nausea. So that's *Frasier*, *Friends* and Larry David . . . all ruined. The effect is so pervasive, the strength of the conditioned response (we did do a lot about those Pavlovian mice at school) to the chemotherapy regime is such that even typing these words I feel the familiar, and not welcome, heaving of my stomach, a wave of impending gorge.

I hover, therefore, over my *West Wing* tapes, guarding their separateness, their status as fragile as freshly poached eggs, subject to ruination at the slightest hint of contamination. I won't let anybody play them in the house, or hospital, on any of the days before, after or during a chemo treatment.

So Anthony's been desperately trying to find stuff I'll watch, but not mind never seeing again. This is not the easiest of balancing tricks to pull off – it has to be engaging enough to divert me from the medical treatment, not to mention the inevitable hours of sitting around while drugs are made up, put on hold, taken off hold, blood analysed and so on. But this suitably involving film or TV programme also has to satisfy that internally contradictory requirement: brilliantly gripping, but so dispensable it doesn't matter if it's spoiled for ever after this one viewing. It's a challenge my husband has been embracing with some energy, spending hours searching Amazon's 'recommendations we think you will like based on previous purchases' tab.

It's *Breakfast at Tiffany's* today. I still want to channel hop, and sit mutinously, looking anything but Givenchy *comme il faut*, as the black and white images slide elegantly across my admittedly beautiful and Hepburn-esque Apple Macbook. I am just becoming involved, drawn in by Hepburn's earplugs and eye-mask chic, when I realize Anthony is now fast asleep on the bed. I'm perched uncomfortably on the edge, trying not to unbalance either my husband or the drip in my arm.

I can't wait for the nurse to come back. Ha, just wait till she sees this, I chuckle to myself, husband flat on his back, deep in slumber on my sick bed.

'Oh, poor love,' she starts, and I'm already eating it up. I could so do with an extra dose of sympathy today. 'Poor, poor love,' she sighs again, hand very close to stroking

Anthony, really hovering on the brink, only that might disturb him. 'It's just so hard on the partners, isn't it?'

∽

'Neutropenia – I'm neutropenic but not febrile, neutropenic but I wear make-up every day now . . . I don't even know what neutropenic means . . . finished *Vogue* piece, lucky I'm up all night . . . so constipated . . . just tell the bloody doctors . . .'

It's 2 a.m. I'm in and out of sleep, words bothering my mind like predators of peace. Symptoms: an infected finger and a mouth so full of ulcers I haven't been able to swallow for three days, and couldn't open my mouth to speak to the teachers at Nina's parents' evening, making do with just nodding and smiling instead. Most unnerving of all, a feeling as if every joint in my body has become fragile and will break if I move, like I'm on a string, and the puppet-master's in a bad mood, and trying to smash me to bits.

Morning comes, and so do Tatiana and Milan. In a novel twist on the celebrity/cleaner axis, where the housekeepers of famous folk sell stories to the tabloids, the twice-a-week help (upped to three times on chemotherapy weeks) we have in this house is a couple from Croatia. Milan, immensely tall, a former footballer in his home town, and Tatiana, a Shakespearean beauty. Before they became refugees, they were a pair who never paid for their own drinks – local neighbourhood heroes.

Tatiana's hair fell out during their years in hiding; it's soft and curly now, but, she says, has half the thickness it used to. I can only imagine the magnetism they had in their home town, because glamour still shades their every move; it's like having Cary Grant and Katharine Hepburn come in to vacuum and make everything gleam a couple of times each week. To top it all, their teenage son Vedrun plays one of the Gryffindor school-boys in the *Harry Potter* movies. So Tatiana doesn't just make my house splendid, she also has Grade A gossip to dispense; every snippet of information from the *Harry Potter* studio is as interesting as it is forbidden by contract to be spread. Cancer has its complications, but stopping myself from spilling movie-set gossip into my *Guardian* column is killing.

Some things are non-negotiable though, and having this help has been key during this illness. And more: Tatiana was the only non-family member I let into the hospital. She came with a basket loaded with the foods I long for, armed as she is with her second-to-none knowledge of what actually goes out of my cupboards and into my mouth.

Today is the first time I call the doctors for assistance. Peter Ostler says he'll see me this afternoon, so I pick Elon up from school and he comes with me for the drive to Mount Vernon, not falling asleep, of course, until we pull into the hospital car park. Inside the hospital the nurses try to distract him, while one takes my blood. I say, through gritted teeth and mouth ulcers, 'Just let him see . . .'

Elon's too smart not to know there's a reason for all these people frantically doing comic turns in the effort to make him turn his face away from the interesting stuff being practised on my arm.

My white blood count is 0.3, which, Dr Ostler says,

means I should probably be admitted to hospital right now, this ordinary school-day afternoon, older children due back home in a couple of hours. 'Out of the question,' I say, pointing at Elon. What is he supposed to do, check into the next bed? Make his own way home?

Actually, I'm torn between that desire to slump straight into the nearest, fresh-linened hospital bed, where time stops for a few days, and nothing has to be done, because you just aren't there to do it, and my other driving urge: being the one on whom everything depends.

'If you start running a temperature,' he says, 'come straight back. I'm telling them to expect you.' But he's also said that nothing about my medical state is too critical: reddish throat, yes; infected finger, sure, 'but nothing to drain'; and no thrush on the tongue. So part of me leaves hospital with that satisfying 'huh, I'm genuinely ill' sensation, and the other half is left with that less comfortable making-a-fuss-about-nothing guilt trip.

Over the next few days, everything clears up. I am feeling completely normal, just in time for the second dose of Taxotere. This is the rhythm of these cancer treatments: you slide into hospital, get drugged and begin feeling fuzzy as you leave the ward, then sink into a more violent illness, out of which you emerge almost imperceptibly, so you don't even realize for a day or so that you've stopped feeling ill, except that you're reminded with a jolt because it's time to drive back for the next round of treatment. As the weeks go on, you also get to contend with a new feeling of dread, brought on by the sense of being battered by the relentless bashing back down just when you're up again, like those deeply unpleasant thrillers where they sustain the tension by allowing moments of recovery before they start the torture again.

But for this next dose of Taxotere, Dr Ostler has rustled up something to help me. This time, twenty-four hours after the chemotherapy, I'm given an injection to boost my white blood cells, something called Neulasta.

The liquid in the syringe is growth hormone, I'm told. Highly recommended; for the first time in months, I feel strong, and not like I'm crossing Siberian plains, dragging lead weights round my ankles through the depths of snow.

This turns out to be lucky because on Sunday morning Nina starts vomiting. Ten times by eight-thirty. By nine, we're at Finchley Memorial casualty department, not the nearest to our home, but reputedly the one with the shortest waiting times in their Accident & Emergency section, where, in fact, they keep us waiting just until she starts throwing up over the reception area, and then she is seen straight away. Useful tactic.

Nina does not, the doctor says, have the appendicitis I have been fearing, but stomach flu. So after I get her back home and into our bed, with rehydrating drinks and a basin nearby in case she doesn't make it to the bathroom sink in time, I take Marganit off to her music exam, and Anthony, a greenish tint round the edges, shepherds Elon to a new kindergarten comrade's birthday party. Back home, Anthony barely climbs the stairs – taking the extra flight up to Chloë's room right at the top of our house, because Nina is huddled in our room – before he falls into bed. Sara-Jenny, director of her school musical this year, comes downstairs at two in the afternoon to say she's having to go into school to supervise six hours' extra rehearsing. I don't even have to say anything, I just count to five, before she sinks on the bottom step: 'I think I'm ill, Mum.'

I feel more than well. Powerful, fantastic injection. It is supremely fortunate, really, that I feel this positive about something which is inserted into my body at the point of a needle, because the next two times I need to use it the nurses give it to me in a neat little box – injection 'to go'. Yes, after a couple of practice shots on a heavy-duty, thick-skinned Jaffa orange, I leave hospital with a pre-packed takeaway dose of Neulasta that I am going to self-inject. All I have to do is open the sealed syringe loaded with serum and insert the stuff into my flesh. The nurse tells me, and this is helpful, that it really doesn't matter what angle it goes in, it will still work.

It is a rainy Thursday school-holiday morning, so I make pancakes. By eleven there is just one scoop of batter left, and Elon pops his head round the door to ask for the last pancake to be brought to him before he races back to the television. Chloë is the only one left in the kitchen when I take the injection pack out of the fridge.

I rub ice all over my stomach, which is where the injection is going. I give Chloë one half of the last pancake to take to Elon and eat the other half with my left hand, while I put the needle into my stomach with my right. I can't believe how easy it is to inject, the only slight pause coming when I make the mistake of looking down, realizing I've actually put the needle in and that I now have to pull the syringe out again, but I just close my eyes and do it. I am still licking up drips of maple syrup from round my mouth, and the whole episode is over. This one feat, more than any other, is a sign of how far removed I now am from my former pre-cancer self.

∞

Demob-happy: seven of eight chemotherapies down and, for the first time, I've chucked out the little white pills instead of dutifully swallowing them. Everybody tells you to take control of this illness, but – until this day of mass tablet extermination – I've just done exactly what the doctors told me to, at every stage. 'Taking control' seemed to me to give the cancer too much importance, make it too much part of my life.

But with only one chemo left, I'm going wild. So bye-bye tablets and, hey presto, the constipation vanishes too. Before each treatment the doctors ask you about your symptoms from the last chemotherapy. I've always answered truthfully about every other symptom, but for some deep reason known only to Freud probably – and he's dead – every time they ask about constipation, I've just said airily, no, no, that's not been a problem at all. In actual fact it's been a massive, huge, enormous and ever-looming difficulty. (For what it's worth, I will pass on the fact that taking a notebook into the loo, and writing three A4 pages before exiting, does help . . .)

Anyhow, what with the vanished constipation, and the power-surge from the growth-hormone injection – which according to my insurance bills costs several hundred pounds, even when I squeeze it into my stomach myself – I'm practically skipping into Center Parcs in Longleat, three hours' drive from London, where we have decamped with six of the children. Center Parcs is

that late twentieth/early twenty-first century phenome-
non: a 'holiday concept'. The first one was opened in
the Netherlands by a Dutchman, who built some villas
in a forest, banned cars in favour of bicycles and said
this was the way to combine outdoor activities with
leisure time. Now he has himself not just a concept, but
a company that trades very nicely, thank you, on stock
exchanges across Europe.

It has taken me two weeks – exactly one week longer
than the time we are going to spend in this English
branch of the concept – but I have finally managed to fill
in the form booking everybody into the multi-spangled
activities on offer here, and so, tonight, it's payback time.

I am off to the spa. Sara-Jenny, Marganit and Chloë
tried it out on night one, and came back saying,
'Mum/Dina, you really have to go; you will love it.' Nine
different types of steam rooms, and a pool open to the
night sky. We're here because *Vogue* has a list of the top
twenty spas in the UK, and Longleat's Center Parcs came
in at seventh place. I am, I muse – as I head down the
dimly lighted woodland paths to the farthest reaches of the
concept, where they keep the spa – always amazed at how
I cannot resist reading and absorbing the information in
these magazine and newspaper Top 20 lists, even though
I know full well that I write exactly those kinds of lists two
or three times a year for the *Guardian*, recommending
children's books, and I cannot claim that every name in
the twenty is there because it is superb rather than just
because the exigencies of space demand twenty names.

As I peer ever more desperately, in the ever-thickening
so-much-darker-than-city darkness, at the few signposts

provided for by the Dutch version of concepts, I hear the distant chuckles of friends to whom I'd mentioned the Center Parcs spa, all of whom had looked at me like I was taking the cancer a step too far when I said I'd booked us a week here. Center Parcs has something of an image problem: all that enforced cycling, friends sniggered, and 'Can you see Anthony doing jolly group activities', by which time the laughter was so heaving they barely had breath left for words.

∞

It was as we packed to head off on this week's communion with nature that I suddenly stopped short as I ran round the house slipping a list under each child's door, detailing the stuff I thought each person needed to take. Reading over my carefully thought-out template of instructions for fully independent children, I suddenly stopped sharply with a huge intake of breath, fear in my belly. How could I go to this holiday village with its fabulous, year-round, multi-slide swimming pools, and its top-twenty spa? What did I think I was going to wear? All those days down Bond Street, and neither *Vogue*, nor I, even broached the thought of what the single-breasted wear in a swimming pool.

How did I not remember the mastectomy when I booked this dream midwinter holiday? The whole point of going away to Center Parcs this freezing December was to take the children somewhere they could swim in what the brochures call a recreation of a tropical paradise (something of an exaggeration, it has to be said, when you actually see the swimming domes, as they are called).

And, of course, to get myself some top-twenty physical pampering. I don't know how I forgot the getting-dressed dilemma – maybe swimsuits seemed too far distant in December – but the holiday was booked, the car was started in the driveway, it was too late to do anything about it, other than take T-shirts to wear over a swimsuit, which are in a bag with me as I head to the spa. My hair is a fuzz over my scalp now, with a little curl at the nape, so I think, will I wear a swimming cap? In a spa? But how odd will a bandanna look?

In reception I tick the medical-condition box, and write breast cancer. I show the release letter from Dr Ostler, saying I can 'partake in any activities', and walk through to the changing rooms. Dimmed lighting, piles of towels. I feel a happy normality just walking in and start to undress. There was a time when I was a gym babe, perfectly happy to strip off in communal changing rooms. Again, I catch myself short. I'm really lucky: tonight, for some unexplained reason, this spa is remarkably quiet (one of the reasons it feels quite so luxurious), but even so, I suddenly realize I do not feel like struggling into a swimsuit for the first time in months, and exposing my scarred body to the gaze of strangers.

Funnily enough, the other woman whose eye I catch has very, very cropped hair. Is she post-cancer? Anyhow, I head for a private changing room. The swimsuit looks OK in this dim light. It is an ordinary black one-piece swimsuit with two shoulder straps. It has some nice detailing under the chest and some neat Lycra tucks that do wonders for your shape, all of which is rather lost when you wear a black T-shirt over the top of it all.

Then I take the T-shirt off, and decide I can get away with that too. 'How flat-chested am I?' I chuckle grimly to myself in the mirror. My 34B bust measurement looks fine in a swimsuit, even though one half of that measurement has been decimated. Well, the main point is I can get away with it. I do not look odd, really, at all; at least, I'm not attracting any glances. I wrap a towelling robe around myself, and then, whee, and hurrah for Dutchmen and their nous with marketing, it's all caution thrown to the winds: I even take off the bandanna. It's trendy, I tell the mirror.

I get the last laugh on all the Hendon nay-sayers. The Aqua Sana is replete with enormous chairs to lounge on as you inhale different steam infusions in each area. And as you are lying back and breathing deeply, out of the floor, like giant hookahs, there are these hoses to switch on and douse yourself down with freezing cold water.

It's one of the best evenings I've ever spent. I can see how the Aqua Sana would be much less enjoyable on a crowded night, but it is a fantastically designed area. I leave so revived the next day I go back for some reflexology. What your body cries out for, post-surgery, is massage, the strengthening contact that reaffirms your body is not something from which to shrink, but I can't quite face that exposure just yet. So I limit hands-on pampering to the very edges of my body.

∽

I am on my last dose of Taxotere. My now very greying hair falls out for the second time with this final dose, and I faint climbing up the stairs at home, falling forward and getting a black eye, the shiner, a badge of honour. I have no eyelashes.

My hair is everywhere. That sensation again, like being singed, a frizzing that – is this my imagination? – it feels like I can hear. It's coming out in clumps, drifting down my face, even though the longest strand is barely an inch.

In between the grey it seems to be the same colour as before though; chestnut-brown, I'd say it's called. I hate looking like this – round-faced, jowly (still struggling to lose the seven chemo pounds) and bald.

It was Marganit's parents' evening last night. Her English teacher had radiotherapy and while she's talking about it she starts to cry. My hair is all around, and so is this illness.

I'm tired. Not doing enough exercise. The doctors want me to have a coil refitted, their paramount concern that there be no chance of my becoming pregnant and I realize I need to make that appointment. It's the post-chemotherapy mind-numbness; you hear yourself thinking incredibly slowly. I am a robot; I must make an appointment.

This Shabbat feels like a long day. I look at myself in the mirror, and in my mind I'm saying, 'I cannot bear looking like this.' And I am achey from the Taxotere and tired. I know it will pass, I hear my brain saying, very, very slowly. But I need to drop this extra weight, I repeat again and again to myself. The fatigue of being ill.

After Shabbat goes out and Elon is finally in bed I watch *Cambridge Spies* with Anthony. It's part of the collection of DVDs he keeps ordering – the one-offs that won't be spoiled by chemo. But this leaves me with sad, disturbed feelings all night, the heightened chemotherapy emotions. Then, at midnight, finally sleep comes, and somebody starts a fireworks party. This becomes a really frightening night, the bangs sounding like gunfire, like we're in the middle of a war zone. This is another drug-induced departure for me: fireworks are, or have been, one of my favourite things – if I had to make a top-twenty list, they'd be right up there in the top five, the ones that made it on to the list purely on merit. But the chemotherapy is like one of those evil witches in fairy tales, the kind that make bright red apples poisonous. On these drugs, menace lurks. A brilliant display of colour becomes the enemy at the gates.

Elon wakes at one o'clock, then again at five-thirty. As Anthony starts playing Lego with Elon downstairs at six-thirty I climb into a bath, my default comfort zone. Coming out of the bath, I'm not sure what to do – crawl into bed, or, better I think, go downstairs and say we should all go out to Hampstead Heath for a walk. Get a grip, I hear my mind saying. Walk.

Elon and Anthony are curled on the couch now watching TV, and I do my disapproving, pursed-lips mother look – the one that blames Anthony for saturating our house with television, instead of, say, training for the London marathon during these early-morning stretches. I bark out, 'Come on, I'll get dressed, let's go to Kenwood.' Turning to walk back up the stairs, I fall flat on my face on the second step up. So, in the end, that's what I do with this morning. I faint.

The last thing I remember is Anthony saying, 'Come on darling, I'll help you back up to bed.' Very gentle, very soothing.

Our bare, polished wooden stairs, wide floorboards of a reclaimed timber that is coveted in some circles (and which the children would like to smother with carpet), deliver me one bashed mouth and a blackened left eye. I am back in bed. This is the first daytime, apart from my stay in hospital, that I have spent the daylight hours lying down.

My mother phones from Israel. She tells me she had an operation on her arm last week, on her shoulder. I say I know what it's like, not being able to lift your arm. I am my mother's fifth child. She was thirty years old when she had me. I had only two daughters by the time I was thirty. When I was pregnant with Marganit, my second daughter, I worried a lot about how she would feel second-rate, how it was inevitable she wouldn't bask in the same glow as her older sister. 'How will it be possible for me to love another child as I love Sara-Jenny?' I fretted daily, as Sara-Jenny and I fed ducks in the park. I sometimes describe to the children how, when each one was born, I physically felt my heart expanding, making a new, distinct space for the newest child.

I phone my children, who are at their father's house. 'I need Sara-Jenny,' I say. 'I need help with Elon.'

I need porridge, I say to Anthony. Food will make me strong. Anthony is anxious now, wanting to do the right thing. He tries to make porridge, but comes back up the stairs looking grey, defeated.

Anthony raises Peter Ostler on the phone, who sounds sleepy this early Sunday morning, and asks me whether I can lift both arms over my head. Yes, I say. 'You probably just need to rest,' he tells me. I'm not exactly sure what phrasing doctors could use to be reassuring while at the same time not making one feel like the patient who cried wolf.

In the afternoon Anthony and Elon go out to the Bar and Bat Mitzvah conference, a large, annual marketplace really, a gathering under one roof of every facility one might need to take a twenty-first-century boy into a thirteen-year-old. Theo's Bar Mitzvah is this coming September, and it is our turn to plan this family celebration.

It is the backdrop of this illness, the way the children's lives are an ever-moving escalator. Nina is choosing secondary schools, and has an interview at South Hampstead High, a private school with an arty reputation.

Forty-eight hours after my fall I'm trying to look cool, calm, avant-garde and relaxed in a headscarf and make-up to lessen the impact of the bruising on my face at Nina's interview. There are big, chunky cookies on the table, and mothers sitting around chatting while their daughters are taken away to be examined. As we leave South Hampstead, Nina trips on the worn stone steps, and stumbles headfirst. She is very shaken by the fall, exhausted by the tension of these decision-making days, and she is only smiling to cover her tears. We go to a cafeteria to recoup, before I drop her back at her junior school.

Back home I feel like everything is just too hard at the moment. I put on *The West Wing*.

I have only been home an hour when the phone call comes from Nina's school. The head teacher wants a word. I am lying on the bed, half watching *The West Wing*, half asleep, and the head teacher's words are drifting in and out of my head flaccidly. I'm only hearing the edges of what she's saying: 'Mrs . . . has died . . . this morning . . .' At first I think she is telling me about some teacher, and that she's simply informing all the parents of shocking news. Then her words come into focus, and I understand.

A mother from the school has died of breast cancer. It is the woman who came up to me on Rosh Hashana to say encouragingly that she had finished her treatment, that, 'Look there is life after it all . . .' The school is phoning me because Nina is crying, some child made some comment to her. Do I want to pick her up?

I put the orange cashmere wrap over my long grey coat, the one that looks like something Mary Poppins might wear, and I am lean, chic and impermeable. Nina's class teacher brings her to the gate and I can see her taking in the outlines of my militantly elegant look. Another child has told Nina, 'Don't you know, ninety-eight per cent of women with breast cancer die of it?'

The rest of the week feels fragile, like an egg with fault lines slowly tracing across it; it started whole, if delicate, but the cracks are showing and spreading fast. Soon, everything will crumble. Anthony's mother collects Elon from school one afternoon to give me additional rest-time. I feel uneasy when she doesn't phone, as she usually does, after picking him up, calling to say he's fine and discuss their plans for the afternoon.

But I tell myself to stop being silly, and just enjoy the extra couple of hours' peace and quiet. Also, to take advantage of the chance to walk home from school with Nina, a chance to talk, without Elon, who only goes to school half-day so ordinarily comes with me to pick up his sisters, jumping up and down. But instead I end up picking a fight with her, and she is in tears again when we reach the top of the road.

Then Myrna phones at three-thirty to say she'll be bringing Elon back late, that he'd had a fall at school and was quite upset when she collected him, but he's fine now, and watching a film. I'm really shaken when I see him at five o'clock – he must have crumpled straight on to the playground gravel, and is badly bruised.

That night I feel like bed is the only safe place, that if any of us moves off our mattresses we will splinter into a thousand pieces.

By the following Monday, which is mine and Anthony's sixth anniversary, my come-back hair is once again, thanks to the Taxotere, left behind wherever I have been. The regrowth has been so minimal, the barest fuzz; but, fallen out, it feels like a lot. Elon and Anthony are both running temperatures, and Anthony is on his first day of what will be a week in bed. By Wednesday, Marganit has flu and asks if there's any chance of chicken soup.

12. The Home Run?

It's the home run, and I am flat on my back again. My arms are over my head and three people are marking me up with felt-tip pens. This is radiotherapy, which is the last stage of treatment the doctors have outlined for me. The people are concentrating intensely, so they make no eye contact with me and limit communications to, 'No moving at all, please, no blinking if possible, very sorry, no coughing.' It takes them about half an hour to process each patient, and the waiting room is crammed.

They are colouring on me even though they have already marked me with tattoos, freckle-sized black ink marks. Tattooing is forbidden under Jewish law, and so, at my first radiotherapy appointment, when you fill in many consent forms, I ask, 'Is there any other way you can do this without tattooing me?'

'That's what everybody asks,' the smiling radiographer says. I'm confused, I don't know whether this comes under the catch-all exclusion in Jewish law – 'necessary for saving life' – that overrides every prohibition. And of course, while I'm having this internal Halachic discussion, the ins and outs of the Jewish legal system, it's to shut out the overriding image: finding myself, a Jewish woman, razed of hair, about to be tattooed.

A long time after this day in the hospital, I do manage to ask my father, head of a rabbinical seminary in Israel, about being tattooed for radiotherapy. 'Why should Jews be tattooed?' he says. He tells me that in Israel they use semi-permanent marking.

But this day, I am in a windowless room in the basement of the Royal Free Hospital's radiotherapy department. The ominous feelings begin as the assistant takes me down the stairs – it feels like a bunker. I cheer myself up by saying it's like the office given to Ainsley Hayes, the blonde Republican Associate White House Counsel, in The West Wing – to test her mettle she is assigned to the boiler room, hundreds of miles from the important offices.

I'm brought quickly back to my own life by this woman with her pink-striped hair and a clipboard saying, 'Now you know, of course, you mustn't get pregnant.' The sign on the way in to the radiotherapy unit has a picture of a pregnant mother with a speech bubble coming from her expanded stomach, saying, 'Tell us if I'm in there, Mum,' a warning that is repeated down the side of the poster in thirty different languages.

'So you're not happy, but you'll have the tattoo marks?' the radiotherapy nurse is saying to me. And she adds, shaking her head in a satisfied way, 'Yes, that's what everybody says.' I simply sign the form.

All I ask is, 'Does the tattoo hurt?' I know a bit about tattooing, you see. Years back I wrote a magazine article about a three-day event in Dunstable, a grim town: 'The

Tattooing and Body-piercing Convention'. It was the early nineties, before studded people were common-place, and folk came from places where body-piercing was outlawed to pay hefty sums of money here. What struck me, apart from the white faces and spurting blood, was how child-friendly the convention was. It was a family affair, people brought their kids, and the small babies were enchanted by the inked-in bodies, and the often quite large, shiny bits and bolts dangling from human flesh on display.

'Oh, it's nothing like as bad as having blood taken,' the radiotherapist is saying to me. 'I'd be surprised if it's worse than having a splinter taken out.' Another friendly smile, as she asks, 'How are you with needles?'

They are comparing angles. A red laser line criss-crosses my body. Behind me, vertically, there is a giant 360-degree circle and they are measuring against the cor-responding circle on the floor. I am the point of a compass, and these people are conductors of radiation.

The men have warm hands, but the women's hands are freezing. 'We have warmer hearts,' one of the women says, and giggles. One of the men has a bad stammer, and another has only half an arm – he and I are the maimed in this room – but he's so friendly, so skilful, so easy, it's three sessions down before I realize it is his stump he is using to shift me the infinitesimal amounts into the exact line required before the machine is started: 'I'm ante', 'I'm post', 'I'm at point-six-five', 'Say when' and 'Happy?' are the phrases these people use. The consultant radiothera-pist, the one in charge, looks intently at my chest, nods, and says yes, put the ball bearings here. Ball bearings?

When they finish the calculating, they say, 'OK, starting now.' And then they flee the room, running, not walking, just before they press the button that starts the whirring. When they return, I ask them why, if they spend all that time making those intricate measurements so the radiation will only get the exact space on my body and not venture beyond the marked-out angles, why do they run like tigers are upon them when the machine comes on? They smile but do not answer – no talking yet – so I begin writing mental lists in my head.

Five Things About Which I Feel Benign

1. Emla cream. You put it on before injections – the blood tests, the drug infusions – and the area is numbed. You have to remember to apply it, though, about half an hour before the procedure, and then you don't feel the needles. My friend Chany, a doctor, living through the worst of personal times, somehow finds the mental and emotional space to tip me off about this bit of medical know-how.

2. My private health insurance company, Standard Life. This will sound contrived, but it's the truth. The very night before this all began, I said to Anthony, 'Why on earth do we need private health cover? We never go to the doctor!' In the event, the insurance company has covered each treatment, without delay.

3. The astonishing Jane, receptionist of this department. Completely unflappable, completely helpful,

never, ever making you feel like you're imposing. She has her pen in one hand, one eye on the computer, and she always waves at people as they come in. She has surreal conversations: 'It's hard to speak to him because he's deaf, and he only speaks Hungarian.'

There is a model of medical secretary/receptionist who hides extreme impatience and discourtesy with patients behind a plaque that declares: 'RUDENESS TO THE STAFF WILL NOT BE TOLERATED'. Jane could be excused the odd bit of short temper. She presides over a radiotherapy department which appears to be processing lines of people all day long, every fifteen minutes, judging from what I can see in the waiting room, and all these people have had to negotiate the atrocious under-provision of car parking in this hospital. But she never once says anything about rules; in fact, I watch her frequently helping people bend the car-parking strictures so they can make their appointments on time. It is not just patients who appreciate her; doctors pass to and fro, coming to her with administration problems, leaving them behind at her desk, during the time I spend in the radiotherapy waiting-room chairs.

4. The radiographer, Yann. He remembers my name, and gives me these cool geloid squares to put on the sore radiated skin. The gel stops the skin from discolouring, he says, and tells me to hold it on the area while I'm reading or watching television.

I stall on number five because one of the radiographers has just put her clipboard down on my stomach. I'm lying so still, she thinks I'm a desk. So now it's Things About Which I Feel Quite, Quite Malignant:

1. Doctors who call breasts 'boobs'.
2. Most other human beings. People, I've learned, love a victim. Because I look well, because I won't wear my illness on my face, women come up to me saying stuff like: 'So-and-so has this, but of course not like yours; she really has cancer.'
3. People who say, 'Surviving?' in an attempt at confronting illness with bonhomie.
4. This freezing-cold radiotherapy room. The radiotherapists say the room will warm up – the treatment is daily – then someone lets slip that 'Haven't you been told, the machines need to be cold to work.'
5. The weight gain from the steroids. The struggle to keep moving, although my joints have grown stiff, and hunched. They have aged me before my time; it's the menopause apparently.
6. Jane the receptionist (again). How humourless she is. One of the men sitting in the waiting room says to her, 'Alice and me, we'll have a cup of tea each.' Jane looks up, frosty. Alice says, 'He's joking.' And he says, 'Full of life, me, never down in the mouth even when they was shooting at me.'
7. The geloid things. These flabby, see-through cushions packed with gel that you keep in the fridge, but which just don't work, even ice-cold. My skin is

so, so, so itchy. The worst patch is on my upper
arm, but when I show it to 'them' they say they're
not even targeting that area . . .

The longer I lie here the worse everything looks.

It's the home run, and I drive myself back from hospital these days. A woman phones to say she is writing an
MA on post-mastectomy dressing, and can she interview
me. And I make pancake mix because it is Nina's birthday.

. I also start trying to find out where I can buy a punchbag for Marganit's birthday, which is just three weeks
away. Three or four trips to the sports shop later, and it
turns out you can order them online. But buying a
punchbag is the least of it; the real challenge is how you
attach it to the ceiling.

It's an established part of the chemotherapy blur how
we have had builders in the house on and off for long
months now. There's been a man building cupboards in
Marganit's room since the early autumn. Ordinarily this
would have me spitting tacks, fuming and furious at the
ludicrously slow pace of work. But although I briefly lose
my cool when he puts the 'built-in' cupboards in the
centre of the room, rather than in the alcoves for which
they were measured, once November passes and he
agrees to redo the cupboards in the form in which they
were originally ordered, I barely notice autumn becoming winter, and then turning slowly into spring, and the
builder still having just one cup of tea, milk and two
sugars, every day.

In the back of my mind, very far back, I can remember

a chap from a kitchen firm saying to me once, with some bemusement, 'I have the impression, Dina, you're the kind of person who's used to things being done very fast.' Yes, once I was the kind of person who could get English builders to install an entire kitchen (and that's a kosher kitchen, mind – two sinks, two sets of virtually everything, for milk, and for meat dishes) in six weeks.

Now I'm the kind of person who's pathetically grateful that the builder I employed last year for a minor job is still in the house now Marganit's birthday has come round, so I can ask him how you hang a punchbag from a ceiling. In case you're thinking of doing this, you have to get another guy, different branch of building altogether, to come round and have a look, and go up in the attic to check ceiling joists, and then he makes an ugly hole in the ceiling, and buys the right metal chain to attach the punchbag.

You know what amazes me about all this, though? It's that the punchbag arrives to our house in a matter of days – click, click on the Internet and this heavy sausage as tall as a man arrives at my front door – and this punchbag, in its wrapping, sits in the front hallway for twelve days until Marganit's birthday . . . and she never even notices it, though she walks in and out of that front door every single day. Having cancer treatment can sometimes make you feel like your senses have been blunted, like you are seeing the world through a thick air bubble, in which you are floating, everything else tuned out. Watching my adolescents, I think the teenage years are not all that dissimilar, mind so preoccupied with friends and schoolwork that you can be sitting right next to the phone when it rings but you won't hear it.

Then, with a jolt, I understand that it's not them, it's me. I don't even realize how locked inside this illness I have become. The nights are always interrupted, phantom aches in my legs, sunburned skin from the radiotherapy. I fall into a dead sleep, too early, then wake at two or three to pace the darkened stairs.

One midnight the phone rings too many times and wakes me up. Sara-Jenny is downstairs and I storm into the kitchen, bleary-eyed and angry, so I don't even notice her white face. 'Please tell your friends not to phone the house so late, they can call your mobile, can't they?' I say, stiff and cold.

'Sorry, Mum,' she says, too mildly.

I fall back into bed, haul myself through the next day, and it's not until she comes home from school that she tells me she broke up with her first boyfriend last night; the late-night rings were comfort calls from girlfriends.

Radiotherapy is a daily routine. For these five weeks of treatment I make my way to the Royal Free Hospital in Hampstead, Monday to Friday. It has to be done every day to be effective, although for some reason this doesn't apply to weekends or, indeed, any public holidays.

I've opted to have radiotherapy at the Royal Free, because it is closer to home than Mount Vernon, where Peter Ostler works. Driving back and forth to Mount Vernon is two hours; it takes fifteen minutes to reach the Royal Free from Hendon. Not including parking time.

If you are having radiotherapy you are given a special parking permit by the radiotherapy department. This entitles you to use one of the six designated parking spaces for radiotherapy patients. Most days there are some fifteen people sitting in the waiting room at any given time, so that maths doesn't work, and every other parking space has a queue of people. As we become bolder – by, say, day three of treatment – we radiotherapy patients start parking right in front of the building (with Jane's tacit compliance), on the lines painted in screaming yellow and marked with the words, 'For Ambulances Only'.

This building makes me obstreperous. It's the first time I've walked through double glass doors bearing the sign, CANCER TREATMENT CENTRE. The first day I drive up to it, I get a shock when I read the words, and have to force myself through the wide entrance, shaking off a superstitious feeling, like making myself walk under a ladder. It's the first time, somehow, that I have walked through a hospital door with the word 'Cancer' emblazoned on it. I realize my feeling of horror is illogical – did I think, for example, that I had an illness called 'Garden Hospital' or was I under the impression I was suffering from a strain of 'Mount Vernon NHS Hillingdon Trust'? So yes, kind of stupid to mind really, but I do.

It's one of the ways I keep the cancer at bay, I guess – by not really believing it is anything to do with me. Until it's named, I don't really take it on board. Funny that. I often say to other mothers how ludicrous our children's teachers are when they try to disguise from the children what level they are at; streaming the children, without admitting that is what they are doing. So the brightest group are called 'Oak', the middling ones are called 'Maple' and the laggards are in 'Pine'. The children always know, I'm fond of saying, you might just as well call the groups clever, average, stupid. But here I am, eight months into my treatment for Stage 3 breast cancer, and I very nearly burst into tears because for the first time in this illness I have to park outside a building which has 'Cancer' engraved in black letters on a dirty-white metal door-front.

Two weeks into the radiotherapy and I claim my seniority in this exclusive club by parking right in front of the door now – not even attempting to wait for one of the six assigned spaces to become free. Even though I am a Hendon driver, a species known for their toughness on the roads, and also a veteran of the school run, another extreme challenge for those on wheels, the fight over the six parking places reserved for radiotherapy patients is too much even for one as hardened as me.

The waiting room is full as usual, and the daytime television is on in the corner of the room. It's a home makeover programme, and I watch with the usual bleary-eyed fascination as they do a whole house between breakfast and lunch. This is almost the most demeaning part of the radiotherapy experience: knowing that at my own home the builders have been working on the same set of cupboards for over eight months now (but who's counting) and day after day in this waiting room I'm presented with evidence that mansions can be built in an afternoon.

Then it's time to go into the little cubbyhole to change into the back-opening green gown, and carry your little pile of clothes with you like an evacuee, into the screened-off area where you will be radiated.

On the couch I quickly fall into position, hands over head and no moving while the three or four radiotherapists make their minute adjustments. I admire their infinite patience, how painstaking they are, even as I resent their concentration that somehow excludes me as a person.

When it's over – and it's a painless procedure, radiotherapy – I dive back in the cubbyhole to switch into my own clothes. In the mirror I can see the marks that nobody has bothered to erase from my chest. Some days they are blue, some days they are black. They look like the kind you'd mark on a dressmaking pattern: four running stitches and two crosses.

And then back out into the car park. As I reach my car, a woman jumps out at me: 'Can I have your space, please?'

'Yes, sure,' I say. But then, as I'm behind the driving wheel, car started and ready to pull out, as if from nowhere – or nowhere that I saw – suddenly three cars are coming towards me, menacingly, each one with serious intentions on this space that I've already blithely, not to say graciously, endowed elsewhere. This is too hard. 'I've promised it,' I mouth, 'to that woman in the blue car over there.'

'We were here first,' all three other drivers mouth right back at me, very loud and clear, even though we all have our car windows tightly closed.

Elon is at kindergarten in the mornings only, so although the actual radiotherapy treatment is only fifteen minutes long, the combined trip, waiting time and treatment take up the whole child-free space. But, week three of the radiotherapy, and he is, finally, well and truly weaned. This morning he climbed into bed and, pointing to my breast, said, 'Why do you have these? These bumps?' Then he explored further, and I could see him registering that yes, there was only one bump in fact. And then, without waiting for me to say anything, he answered his own question. 'I had milk there when I was two,' he said. And grinned. No longing, no sadness, just a chuckle and he snuggled down.

I have my own questions about life. 'Why do you all run out of the room?' I ask the most approachable of the radiotherapists again. I never had an answer the first time I put the question.

'Oh,' he says, 'we have to leave the room, or we'd lose our jobs.' Then, his intense calculating and concentrating and measuring completed, he explains, 'It's because x-rays have unpredictable paths. So while we take the utmost care to ensure the x-ray will only hit the targeted area, we can't be sure.'

The end of my radiotherapy coincides with the run-up to the biggest Jewish holiday of them all, Pesach, normally a feat of organization, household disruption and meal-planning. Instead of which we take off for a two-week hotel stay in Israel, which involves nothing more strenuous than packing bags, preceded by an appointment with Mr Al-Dubaisi, something in the nature of a signing off.

'You are looking at me like you don't believe me,' he says to Anthony during one of their man-to-man chats across the desk, me in the chair to the left, nearest the window. 'But I'm telling you the truth. I've been doing this for many, many years. And I am telling you that we often have women coming to us [claiming breast cancer] because they don't like their breasts. They want surgery. And then,' he says, 'we have the women whose lumps are so big by the time they come to me, I cannot believe it.'

Anthony is worrying, asking the surgeon what care will be taken of me now that I have finished the prescribed series of treatment: the chemotherapy, the surgery, the radiotherapy.

Last night, sitting at the table, Anthony suddenly asked, 'How do you feel about all this breast cancer?'

Surprised, I laughed. 'What do you mean?' I replied.

'You're so insouciant about everything,' he said. And then, he adds, dispirited, 'I can't get rid of this cold. I've had it for too long now.'

Daydreaming out of the consulting window, as Anthony and Mr Al-Dubaisi talk on, my mind is stewing with other problems. We have not one but two independent bra emporiums within twanging distance from where I live.

The fitters at Rigby & Peller's – corsetiers to the crowned – famously say they can tell your bra size as soon as you walk through the door. You think that's clever? The women in Frank's and Madame Leiberg's can tell, from the doorway, exactly which of their competitors gave you that misshapen thing you're wearing that is completely spoiling the line of your clothing, dear, if you don't mind me mentioning it.

It is to Madame Leiberg's that I go as I realize that no way am I going to be able to get by in a swimming pool, or on a beach, without some help. What worked in the muted light of a spa in England – just wearing a swimsuit, and to hell with it – simply won't pass muster under the vivid Mediterranean sun. Also, if you actually want to swim, I've discovered, you have to fill out the gap some way, because otherwise the water does, sloshing in and out of my swimsuit.

As I step through Leiberg's door, the kind that chimes as you push it, another customer is telling a 'you wouldn't believe what happened to me in Frank's' story. I eschew such desperate attempts at ingratiating myself with the last remnants of the Austro-Hungarian empire who deign to staff this joint, and just say straight out, 'I need your expert help.'

'Oh, sounds serious,' the assistant replies, making light of it.

'Yes,' I say, 'I've had a mastectomy.' Her face quickly shows that this is grave indeed, but she still leaves the curtain wide open as she sashays in and out of the changing room to bring me different solutions to try out.

They have the swimsuits (ones with pockets ready to have foam fillers sewn in) and they have the neutral-coloured shapes to slip inside. This is exactly what I've resisted so far, these phoney solutions that really rub your face in what has happened to your body, and I'm practically crying as I pay, when out of the corner of my eye I catch this reluctant teenager who's been hauled in by her mother, and the sales assistant is saying, 'Do your friends wear padding then, dear?' And that seems worse.

Even with the foam insert brilliantly stitched into place, the scar is still visible, so I wear a T-shirt over the top of my swimsuit. In any event, in sunlight, I need the extra cover, because the area treated by radiotherapy cannot be exposed.

The foam inserts hold up well in Israel. As an unexpected side-benefit, wearing a T-shirt over your swimsuit does also render you invisible poolside. Everybody, from ancient Russian men playing cards, to swaggering French lawyers, jostles me, or refuses to make way, as I move about the place. It's like suddenly waking up to find yourself the see-through heroine of an Anita Brookner novel.

It's not that I have ever exactly been eye-candy – a phrase the magazine *Time Out Tel Aviv* seriously overuses – but you know, given exactly the right shade of acid-green swimsuit, and on a good day, I could get noticed. No longer.

Still, I'm not complaining. I'm in an ice-cold saltwater pool on a blisteringly hot day, looking out at the sea just below me, windsurfers bright on flecked waves. It's great to be by the sea in Israel, not to be able to see any borders at all in this country where you are always aware of the edges of nationhood, except here, just water stretching as far as the eye goes.

So my mind is far away and Elon finally gets the chance to do what he's been attempting all holiday. No mean feat this one. He's managed to swim right up to me, pull my T-shirt off my shoulder, reach in and yank down the straps of my swimsuit, to expose Mr Al-Dubaisi's undoubted craftsmanship to this glitzy, holidaying crowd, as he announces triumphantly, 'That's the flat one, Mummy, of the ones I used to drink from when I was a baby.'

Boy, I sure do have that gorgeous lifeguard looking at me now.

13. The Knowing Infant

In my mind, Mr Al-Dubaisi (his first name is Muhamed, but it might as well be Mr) is the father. This is down to his manner, rather than his age: he has a two-year-old child, he is a young man himself really, but he has a formality which makes him seem older. He is the surgeon, the one who wields the knife, so maybe I see patriarchal echoes – Abraham, preparing to sacrifice his son. Who knows? The fact is, he has been calling me Dina ever since our first meeting, the night he diagnosed the breast cancer.

Peter Ostler, the oncologist, the one who decides the chemotherapy regime, is the son. He phones me and says, 'It's Pete', and generally calls me 'you'. And, though I could be wrong about this, I occasionally notice some jockeying for position between surgeon and oncologist, the odd remark that hints at competing superiorities, which fits the father-son dynamic.

Glenda Kaplan, the consultant radiologist – who confirms on a screen what the others are thinking – she, of course, is the mother, even though she always calls me 'Mrs Julius', my married name. Soft-looking, she bustles about in a slightly scatty manner, only becoming fully focused as she watches what her scanner reveals on the screen.

Because she is the mother, she is the one who acknowledges the fact that I have been writing about this process from the start – and because she is the mother, her asides reveal she's pleased I'm doing something useful with my time, but should I really be writing about stuff I'm not qualified to discuss?

It is, above all, infantilizing to have a life-threatening illness. Just under a year now since I leapt – in one doctor's appointment – from being me, to being labelled with this mortal sickness that makes everybody lower their voice before they get to the end of the word: can-cer, so the second syllable comes out in a reverent hush.

No other time, as an adult, are you so wholly reliant on other people's knowledge and expertise. Summer a year ago I didn't know what chemotherapy was, except it was a word loaded with fear and loathing. 'Turns out it's something they inject,' I wrote the day of my first treatment. As for the chemotherapy regime: four doses of one drug, then four doses of another, more experimental and hugely more expensive – well, this was opinion-taking well beyond my remit. How on earth was I supposed to assess the pros and cons of one chemotherapy treatment over another? At no other time in my life has my survival depended on being in the hands of the right carers. I am the knowing infant.

For a year or so now I have been living like a cog in others' wheels, simply following instructions, just turning up. My veins coursing with drugs, my body operated on and left single-breasted, myself, lying on a machine alone in a room pinpointed by radiation. I am at the end of all these treatments now: chemotherapy, surgery and radiotherapy all finished. As abruptly as the doctors pick you up, shattering your life into shards of space between appointments and treatments, so they suddenly let you go, back into the community, the grown-up world.

∞

I sit one morning in the café in Hampstead, near the Royal Free Hospital that I frequented daily on my trips to the radiotherapy machines. My head is uncovered. I have hair. The liberation of it, and also the coldness of it. I'm sitting in a café, and my head feels cold because I'm not wearing a bandanna or a beanie. There's a breeze, and my hair – such as it is – is standing on end, so like one of those dolls, where the netting on the scalp shows through, I can feel where my hair is attached to my mind.

I feel both more free, and less intact – like the world can see in to me somehow, in a way it couldn't when I was sheathed in scarves.

The hair is still so short, I can just about pinch a piece between forefinger and thumb. It is, though, long enough to colour. My hair fell out and grew back twice this past year, but this last time it came back grey, a grim colour. 'I won't be grey, I will not be grey, I don't do grey.' I'd find myself conjugating the horrors of grey, without even realizing I was talking to myself.

The hairdresser looks at me tentatively. 'Obviously you've checked this is OK to do?' she asks. No, I admit, I haven't.

'Oh well, this is all completely organic, purely vegetable,' she says. That's fine, I say. As long as it gleams brown like conkers, touched with autumn golds.

I collect Elon from kindergarten with my new hair. 'Oh, I've never seen you without a hat,' another mother says chattily.

'Your hair's short,' a schoolboy says.

Mutinously, under his breath, Elon says, 'But she's hair is going to grow.' Elon's grasp of grammar is still in the early stages, but his firm ownership of me is completely established, his male prerogative to defend me in the playground. Later that week, after the first few days of my new hair, Nina texts me: 'pls, Mum, can u wear hat 2 pik me up. Xxx.'

I head back to the Garden Hospital – the small private clinic very near my home where I had my mastectomy – for a post-treatment mammogram, one of the letting-go rites. My skin where my breast used to be itches incessantly from the radiotherapy. I go through pots of aqueous cream, reaching for the tub, slipping my hand under my shirt to rub cream in even when there are people around. So I'm not looking forward to leaning my right side on to the mammograph, and then I realize – oh, of course, they won't be x-raying that side. Some five months after the operation to remove my breast and I can still be surprised that it's not there any more.

I haven't seen Glenda Kaplan for some months, not since the original barrage of x-rays to diagnose where cancer was in my body, and long before my column in the *Guardian* about this illness began to appear.

I have a sense that the nurse has been told I'm a journalist – she is very solicitous as she takes me to the x-ray room, all the while watching my face warily – and that it's because I described in the *Guardian* how uncomfortable it is to be mammographed. A machine designed by men, I wrote.

The mammogram is clear, Dr Kaplan tells me straight away. It is one of the maternal things about her – she gives good news at once, never waiting for protocol. Although, she says, 'I'm worried about saying anything – because I know it'll appear in a paper in a few months.'

She's only half-joking. A bit later she says, 'Well, I did like your *Vogue* piece, about the clothes. I thought that was good.' I don't think it's my imagination that she's saying it's all right for me to write about clothes, but stay off the medicine.

One of the surprises of this past year is realizing – from their reactions – how very rare it is for doctors to read descriptions of what it feels like to be treated by them. They don't know, for example, how various procedures hurt. It gives them a detachment that is almost tangible.

It is as I come out of the cocoon stage, doctors letting go, that I come bang up against a dilemma that must take all the detachment any doctor can muster. What do you do when you know there's a life-saving drug available, but only the patients who can afford it can have it?

Almost without realizing, my strength is coming back. Instead of slumping, one evening Anthony and I actually go out, to hear Michael Douek, senior lecturer and consultant surgeon, speak about 'latest developments in breast cancer'.

He's radiating energy, and he's not mincing his words. He says there are new results out, about a drug called

Herceptin, which patients who are Her-2 positive should be demanding, though it hasn't been approved in the UK yet.

I hear Michael Douek long before Herceptin penetrates the British media. Something about his very definite manner, his disparaging of cost considerations, the way he says, 'Whatever it costs I tell my patients to get it', all coincides with a memory I have from the early days of diagnosis.

I remember Peter Ostler telling me I wasn't oestrogen positive. 'But that's the good kind, oestrogen positive, isn't it?' I'd said then.

'Well,' he replied, 'don't think of it like that, it just means Tamoxifen doesn't work for you.' And he'd added, 'Your tumour is Her-2.'

The day after hearing Michael Douek I phone Mr Al-Dubaisi to ask about Herceptin. Part of the infant-nature of being a patient with a mortal illness is that you don't really take decisions – what point is your decision-taking unless you are a specialist in the field? Anthony laughs hollowly these days about what he calls the 'charade' of me choosing mastectomy over lumpectomy. 'There never was a choice,' he says. 'From the second you walked into the doctor's office, the size that tumour was, it was always mastectomy for you.' He's right. The doctors were creating an illusion of choice, on the assumption that autonomy is helpful for cancer patients.

However, the introduction of Herceptin is so new, this time my phone call is crucial. And yet it isn't really medical reasons that are behind my asking for Herceptin. If I analyse it, I know that part of the reason I have made this call is that I have a sense of insecurity, of loss, now that my life is quite devoid of the roster of doctors' appointments that I've complained about so much this past year. Phoning to ask about Herceptin is a way of reinstating contact with the doctors – a bit like reaching out to get the security blanket of nonstop medical treatment back again.

Whatever my motives, it is my asking for Herceptin that triggers my doctors into getting it for me. And the fact that I asked for it so soon is pivotal; it only works taken this fast after the arsenal of other treatments doctors wield against cancer, the axis of three: chemotherapy, surgery, radiotherapy. In fact, in the States, they're giving Herceptin simultaneously with the first doses of chemotherapy. I finished my last chemotherapy at the end of January, the last dose of Taxotere. It is now May, so I am still within the six-month margin the doctors believe is required for Herceptin to be effective.

There are, though, tests I need to undergo before the final decision about whether I should take this drug or not is taken. I have also asked the doctors about having an MRI. 'Ah,' Peter Ostler says when I ask, 'you've obviously been reading again . . .'

He says he'll organize the MRI, but phones back later on when I'm in the park with Elon to say he's made an appointment for me to have some kind of heart test. I can't hear exactly what he says the test is called, but he says he needs the results of this test before I see him to decide about Herceptin. One of the side effects of the wonder drug is that it can damage your heart, information to which I pay the scantiest attention.

It's a mild afternoon, and I'm wearing the same shirt

for the third day running, deep aubergine crinkled velvet from Marks and Spencer's, of course. Summer is coming, which is great, but all I can think about is what I will wear all summer long? I want to wear T-shirts, I mutter fiercely. I notice myself hunching one shoulder these days to compensate for my imbalance. I even take out the despised 'cumfie' and wear it for an afternoon under a black T-shirt with a black skirt – my old uniform – and feel normal for a few hours. But by the end of the experiment my skin is sore – the area that has been radiated remains extremely tender and dry – and I go back to my sleeveless cotton vests, with layers on top.

Mr Al-Dubaisi phones to intone that 'the MRI is not standard, but since you are young, we will arrange it for you'. And about Herceptin he says, 'Yes, you should have it. I don't think there is anything wrong with your heart.'

I am dismissive of heart anxieties, anxious to start the new drug as quickly as possible. My heart is completely fine, I tell the doctors, who look amused when I say this kind of thing.

My life is now comfortably restocked with medical appointments again, and I'm stressed out about how much time it's all taking, so I end the day by yelling at both Sara-Jenny and Marganit about the state of their rooms. I feel overtired and overweight, deep in cancer-mode.

14. Wonder Drugs

As well as the MRI and heart scans I've let myself in for, I'm also having gene testing, to see whether the kind of breast cancer I'm carrying is genetic.

Before the appointment I've had to send my parents a form to fill out with details of which of my relatives have had any kind of cancer. My father faxes the details back to me: his brother's skin cancer, my grandmother's breast cancer, my two great-aunts' breast cancer, my grandfather's stomach cancer, my uncle's brain tumour, amongst several others. 'Our family's riddled with cancer,' I say to my father on the phone.

'Oh no,' he says, 'not really.' He calls cancer, 'this condition'.

The geneticist at Northwick Park has the errant communication skills of medical folk (is it their genes or their environment?) and she manages in our twenty-minute talk, and despite her soft and gentle manner, to scare the wits out of me about the possibility of my cancer being genetic. Genetic cancer is more aggressive, she explains, and should the test prove positive there'd be an argument for removing my womb, my ovaries and my second breast. 'Am I being clear?' she asks kindly. I stare at her blankly.

She asks some questions about my family history. Was my Uncle Peter treated for his skin cancer? I have no idea, I tell her. Then she asks, 'How's your science?' and I shrug. She does a drawing of an oval, and tells me that is a cell, and then she pulls out a diagram showing twenty-two pairs of chromosomes, plus, down the bottom, the X-chromosome.

I'm stressing about whether she's going to ask me any minute which is the male, the X or the Y, or is it some combination, for the life of me I can't remember, so I nearly miss her next words: 'Thirteen and seventeen are the guilty ones,' she says, pointing to the two pairs of little black wiggly lines on her laminated sheet. 'They can carry BRCA1 and BRCA2.' Ah, I know this. BRCA1 and 2, the breast-cancer genes.

I'm just about recovering from feeling like I'm going through a biology exam for which I haven't crammed when she tells me she has to take some blood. There is the by now standard palaver with my veins, me clenching and unclenching my fist, while the person trying to get the blood taps insistently up and down my arm while heaving sighs and making 'tsk, tsk' noises. 'As you can see, my eyes are on stalks today, I've got terrible hay fever. I think I'll get someone else to take your blood,' the geneticist says.

A nurse comes in, tells me she's from Central Africa, where she trained. The practical side of nursing is better taught in Africa, she says, because nurses have to work in every department, from cancer to maternity, but the theoretical, she says, sighing, is much more intensive in the UK. 'I'm no good with computers,' she laughs. Over the year of treatment I've realized I'm always happier, and I physically relax, when the African nurses appear. They are naturally warm, not wearing their friendliness like a surgical mask, and their touch is easy. 'Ah, these are a bit elusive,' the nurse chuckles, in that rich way the African nurses have, but she gets the huge vial of bright-red blood.

The blood is going to be sent off, and will take some time to come back, I'm told. It will be six to eight weeks at the very least. Also, they won't give me the results when they arrive, over the phone or in a letter. I have to be issued with an appointment to come in and hear the report in person. 'Really?' I say, 'I think that's more anxiety-inducing.' The geneticist makes a face, sort of agreeing, I think, but says this is the protocol and there's no straying from it.

I am home in time for the end of the school day, and that evening I head out again for the MRI scan, which also turns out to require a needle in my left hand. They try my arm first, but comment, 'This has been overused today.' Glenda Kaplan supervises the attempts to put the needle in: 'Don't write about this,' she chuckles, admonishingly. Then, waving her hand over me like a hypnotist, she says, 'You will forget about this . . . you will forget about this . . .'

You have to go face down into the MRI machine, which makes a loud, intermittent grinding noise. So just before you head into it, they hand you earphones and a list of CD titles to choose from. Any residual anxiety from the insertion of the injection is swamped by performance anxiety – what do I choose? Black-Eyed Peas? Elvis Presley? Jazz? Classical? What assumptions will they make about me based on my choice? I stab blindly, and it's Frank Sinatra, which is quite good face down inside an MRI machine – raspy cocktail tones, empowered lyrics.

While I'm sweating over what my musical listening reveals about my personality (to people who are busy gazing deeply into parts of my body I will never be able to access), Anthony has taken Elon to Chloë's school to watch her perform in 'Battle of the Bands', a school musical competition. My mobile rings as I come out of the MRI with the news that Chloë's group have come second – more champagne on ice.

By nine I am back home. Nina, Marganit, Anthony and I watch *The OC*, teenagers through the TV screen. I'm desperate for something to eat, but the kitchen's a mess. I tidy up and find there is chicken soup in the freezer. In two days it is my birthday, but first there is a mammogram tomorrow – absolutely the last of the winding-up rites – and tomorrow night, Madonna is phoning me. Well, put that another way, I have a phone interview scheduled with Madonna, who is publicizing the last of the six children's stories she has written.

As the day goes on I become more anxious about this mammogram than any other procedure I've had, I think. I'm beginning to understand what the doctors mean by saying it isn't useful to give cancer patients checking-up procedures. On the other hand, not having any check-ups is just as bad. Anyhow, Glenda Kaplan says she can see some lymph nodes on the screen, but they're nothing to worry about. So that's OK, then.

All day long Madonna's publicist has been keeping me updated with the details of exactly what time the pop star's phone call will happen. It's moved from 8.15 p.m. to 8.40 p.m. by six in the evening when I head off for the mammogram. When I return home by seven-thirty it's still scheduled for 8.40 p.m., so that's an hour to settle Elon with one more story before sitting poised at my desk. Madonna is phoning from New York. 'I have Madonna for you,' her nice-sounding assistant says at 8.39 exactly.

'Dina?' Madonna says. 'Hi, it's Madonna here. Am I talking to you in London?'

She sounds so young and normal. But our conversation goes downhill from there. I ask her how she, a canny businesswoman, can be involved with the Kabbalah Centre, regarded by the Jewish community as a gathering of charlatans.

'Is it really?' she says, and sounds surprised, which is surprising to me in turn, since I think that's common knowledge. 'Well, you wouldn't think my teachers are charlatans,' she says. 'But they are innocent, naïve, when it comes to publicity.'

We talk for about twenty-five minutes, she draws it to a close, and I have only just begun enjoyably replaying every detail and intonation when the phone rings again. 'Hello,' says a deep male voice. 'Is Anthony there?'

'Sure,' I say, very jaunty, 'who's calling?'

'This is Philip Roth,' comes the grainy reply.

'Oh, wow,' I say, 'this is a really good night for this phone – I've just finished talking to Madonna.'

Roth pauses, then chuckles, and says, 'Surely you don't think I'm a male Madonna . . .'

Thursday's my birthday. Nina's fretting because she went for a haircut at one of the six local hairdressers Hendon spawns, none of whom can cut hair in a way that looks anything other than immediately suburban. Predictably, Nina hates the result. I'm supposed to be going to the hospital for the heart test, which I've now discovered is officially known as a Multiple Gated Acquisition Scan (Muga). I toy with the idea of cancelling so I can take Nina to my hairdressers' to see if they can soften the edges of the extreme chop she's been given. I take another look at the hospital letter detailing the Muga-scan appointment, and on re-reading, realize this scan is a two-injection job.

So that's that decision taken. I phone the hospital, postpone the scan for a week, and take Nina into town instead, where at Fourth Floor – a hairdressers' so good they hide away on the upper floors of a nondescript building so only those in the know can find them – Linda sympathizes with Nina's distress, and snips so tactfully the hair is smoothed into place again.

On Friday Dr Ostler phones to find out why I've missed the appointment and we talk round the question of Herceptin again. He explains once more that I must have the heart tests before I go on the drug, and he explains it will be three-weekly injections. 'Oh,' I say, 'can't it be tablets?' I don't know why, but in my mind I assumed it was oral medicine.

He also says, with only a hint of reproach, that if we're going to decide on Herceptin, we need to start straight away, as its effectiveness is dependent on being given in close conjunction with the earlier chemotherapy.

'Do you have a problem with your veins, or is it just me?' asks the doctor attempting the first of the two Mugascan injections.

'No,' I sigh, 'it's not just you.' I silently grind my teeth and curse – why do they tell me there's a problem, why don't they just get on with it, why, oh, why can't all doctors and nurses learn to be expert at taking blood and administering injections?

After they put the needle in the nurse tells me I'm now somewhat radioactive, and 'mustn't have a young child sitting on my lap for twenty-four hours, or give a close cuddle or hug'. I nod assent, and do the silent cursing of medical profession thing again. 'How's that supposed to work?' as our teenagers would put it. There is a gap in understanding between these doctors and the actuality of my daily life. Just how do you refuse to cuddle a small child after a whole day at school?

I sign a form saying I'm not pregnant or breast-feeding, and feel the familiar wash of sadness. In the playground where I wait to collect Elon the other women are mostly on their second child and just toying with the idea of having a third. I used to say that I don't know how you ever decide not to have more children, how tempting it is to just throw all thoughts of recovering your former self to the winds for another swoop into motherhood – which only gets easier the more times you do it. But these days I don't feel that any more, don't feel at all tempted. I'm too tired.

After the first needle they leave you to wait for half an hour while the radioactive stuff sloshes round your body. The television in the waiting room is broadcasting tips about how to keep your house clean: white vinegar works on telephones apparently, but for mirrors you need to dilute some fabric conditioner.

We make our own tea in this waiting room, from a metal box stuffed with bags, a pint of milk in the small fridge and sugar in a covered bowl. Donations are accepted into another tin, just beneath the sign that warns about the importance of washing hands and MRSA.

Then it's into a gleaming new room for the Muga scan. The walls are a pale purple colour, and the scanner is an enormous piece of white sculpture, which lowers itself down on your prostrate body. The second needle is given now, lying down, and it hurts. I'm needled out.

But then I fall asleep on the x-ray table for the twenty minutes or so it takes to scan my heart, while in the background the radiographer chats in a low hum on the phone.

I wake up and, in a fog, make my way out of the endless halls of this old building, back to the car park where I realize I don't have the two pounds and ten pence I need to raise the barrier that will let me drive away. So this is the day that I find out – exactly a year since I first set foot in this hospital – that, for a mere 50p, there is a machine that will give me tokens I can also use to exit the car park.

The Muga scan out of the way, and clear, Dr Ostler brandishes graphs at Anthony and me demonstrating how the European and US trials have shown that women who are given Taxotere, Adriamycin and Herceptin have better survival chances.

'We were all at Orlando,' he says. 'If you can imagine the conference, two rooms full of five thousand oncologists, and everyone in that room hearing better results from these trials than we've heard for anything recently.'

He pauses expectantly. 'Any questions?' Neither Anthony nor I have anything to ask. 'Oh,' Dr Ostler says, sounding a little disappointed. 'I expected more questions.' He is enthusiastic, wants to relay to us some of the medical excitement and debate about this drug, and we are just sitting, staring at charts delineating the most gradual of descents in their black lines of disease progression, and trying to make sense of it all.

Dr Ostler carries on talking about how Herceptin was being used for more advanced cancer, but how the thrill of this latest conference was finding out that it had an effect on early breast cancer too – cancer that hasn't spread out of the breast. He looks up at us again to see if this dose of exegesis has triggered any analytical questions in our minds.

So I say, 'Uh, does taking Herceptin delay reconstruction?' Bra-burningly bullish about wanting clothes that reflect my new reality, and about giving myself time to adjust to mastectomy, I am becoming ever more open to the idea of just getting my shape back, and can see the end in sight – Mr Al-Dubaisi's imposed deadline of two years, designed, so he's told us, not to allow any chance of the reconstruction being affected by radiotherapy complications.

'Oh, good question,' Dr Ostler says, before adding airily, 'Well, we don't know – we haven't given it before.'

'And can I have some Emla – the numbing cream – before they put the drip in?' is my final stab at an intelligent question about this cutting-edge new drug.

The last ritual before beginning the new treatment – £23,000 for a course of twelve injections – is a set of blood tests. Today's nurse is swift and painless. 'Many people don't do it unless they can *see* the vein,' she says, when I ask how she manages to get the needle in so seamlessly, without the huffing and puffing I've come to regard as routine. 'But it's absolutely OK as long as you can feel it.' More than any other aspect of this illness, I feel real anger at having medical practitioners inflicted on me who just don't have this apparently common-or-garden skill which is nevertheless in short supply: the ability to stick a needle into a vein.

Within days I'm on the first dose of the new wonder drug, a clear fluid, given intravenously. The children do have a question ready: does it make you lose your hair?

The bag of fluid is labelled 'Trastzumatab 530g'. The nurse asks me to confirm my name and date of birth before she starts the transfusion. Behind the next curtain I can hear another woman: 'It's best if I can't see what you are doing,' she is saying quietly. 'All this chemo. It's the first time I've had needles in about fifteen years.'

Another procedure. The nurse has to do an ECG, another test to make sure my heart is ticking neatly. I lie on a tiny bed in a cupboard-sized room. I take off my top and wonder whether these nurses have seen a mastectomy before. They always look.

Then I have tags and cables fastened to me, colour-coded. I feel like I'm a car being jump-started after a battery fault. Red and yellow to left, red and green to right. Next door the woman has now started deep-breathing to ease herself through the injection process.

The tags slip off my aqueous-cream-soaked skin, so the nurse adds sticky tape to keep them on. Then she tells me this is a particularly swanky ECG machine, compared to the one in the last hospital in which she worked.

All rituals out of the way, and I'm in a chair, with a cannula inserted into the back of my hand. 'You're not going to faint on me,' the chemotherapy nurse says. It feels cold as it goes up my veins, and she gives me an out-of-date leaflet about Herceptin to read. 'Herceptin is used to treat secondary breast cancer (breast cancer that has spread to other parts of the body).' The leaflet was written in July 2002. Nobody bothers to tell me the leaflet is out of date, or to say that, of course, Herceptin is being given to me for early breast cancer.

The Herceptin drip lasts ninety minutes. The nurse taps buttons on the stand, like she's setting a burglar alarm. I think about my interview with Madonna, which needs some rewriting. I've been negotiating the price for it with Ian Katz at the *Guardian*. 'Blimey, Dina,' he's emailed me when I ask for more money, 'have you been on one of those tough-talking courses?'

The woman in the next cubicle opens her curtains so we can chat. She's forty, and the only surviving member of her family. Her parents and her sister are both dead. They didn't all die of cancer, she says.

The uproar in UK newspapers and on television and

radio is just starting to roll as women campaign for Herceptin to be available to all. It's the drug that can save a thousand lives a year, they're saying, but is not yet universally available because it hasn't been approved on the NHS, so right now it's being given only to those who can afford to pay for it, or – as in my case – whose insurance companies will put up the money.

The same week in which the newspapers all feature Barbara Clark, a feisty, blonde 49-year-old nurse, launching her battle to be treated with Herceptin, I am back at Mount Vernon, in a chemo lounge waiting for my second dose of this see-through fluid.

I have the usual blood test, and then nothing. I read the papers, and sew twelve nametags into school uniforms. Next term, after the coming summer, Elon will be in uniform: charcoal-grey shorts, a white polo T-shirt, grey socks, heavy black shoes.

Then I realize this is all taking even longer than usual, that there's a silence around me. I figure something is up, and make my way down the corridor to the reception area.

Discomfited faces greet me. Also there is Peter Ostler, looking annoyed. 'I'm so sorry,' the American nurse says. 'This one is three hours past its expiry. I can't give it to you.'

'How did this happen?' Dr Ostler asks.

Behind us, another nurse is disposing of the small square plastic bag, complete with contents, hurriedly shaking the fluid into a square white sink. 'Wow,' I whistle, 'what did that just cost?'

Dr Ostler, who loves figures, started tapping: 'Uh, let's

see, two thousand pounds or so.' The American nurse looks like she is reliving Vietnam.

'God, that's terrible,' she says. 'It came off hold too early.' (In non-medical speak, this translates roughly as, 'The pharmacy took it out of the fridge too soon.')

And then the crucial phrase: 'Are you OK to come in again for it tomorrow, Dina?'

For me, bags of Herceptin can just be flushed down a sink. I'm swimming in the stuff. Elsewhere in England, women are taking court actions, claiming that by denying the drug to all the NHS is in contravention of the European Human Rights Act.

And once again, I hear the echo in my ears. Something Mr Al-Dubaisi said at my last consultation with him. Anthony was fretting. What happens now? How do we know the cancer's gone?

Mr Al-Dubaisi said various things, about how extra scanning can cause more anxiety than reassurance, about the symptoms to look out for – dyspepsia, back pain, unusual headaches – but as we got up to leave the room, he looked over, and he said something I almost didn't catch. 'Dina had a good treatment,' he said. The words hang in the air, and they are haunting. Dina had a good treatment. Not everybody gets the same. It is neither the first, nor the last, time I will hear from doctors that my treatment is 'gold standard', the best, a Sinatra of medical protocol.

15. Recurrence

old has started to tint the trees, and we have new males in our house. The bulging-eyed ones, Scott, Virgil and Allan, enter my life at the same time as Matt, the Healthcare at Home male nurse, who comes round every third Tuesday to hook me up to a plastic bag dripping Herceptin into my veins. I have come through the first few Herceptin treatments without side effects, so – apart from a monthly scan of my heart – I can now have the drugs infusion at home.

He is a huge man, Matt, who wears a single gold earring, and talks of things like 'sharps bins' – it's where you keep your needles – and about how male nurses used to 'fly' but 'we don't fit the public profile anymore'.

Scott is yellow, Virgil's completely orange, but Allan is palest buttercup, with silver streaks. My neighbour, down the road, to whom I have only ever been good and kind – unstinting with the spoonful of baking powder, the cup of sugar, the tablespoon of apricot jam, I remember – pitched up with the colourful newcomers who are about to become such a source of intense anxiety to me I contemplate giving up neighbours for ever. They are a belated gift for Elon's fourth birthday: three goldfish who come to our house in a see-through pale-blue capsule – like a small incubator – carpeted with a thick layer of tiny, irregularly shaped aquamarine gravel.

It is the end of the second summer of this illness. It's bemusing to realize that just fourteen months ago, this was all new and so shocking. Now I'm so blasé, I can have a drip attached to my left arm, and finish off writing table plans for Theo's Bar Mitzvah with my right hand.

Matt arrives in a family-sized car on the Tuesdays he treats me. Against his massive frame, the medical paraphernalia looks like trinkets: the stand for the drip, the cardboard box in which the drug is sealed with heavy tape, the yellow toolbox in which he keeps his other equipment.

He plays water polo, so he's fantastically fit, but he considers himself too large, so he wants to lose weight, and 'the wife' would like it too. You find stuff out about guys, when you're alone in your house with them, and they're sticking needles up your arm.

While the medical side may be routine these days, there is a whole new social etiquette – to me, anyhow – involved in this home treatment. I remember Dr Ostler asking me, at my very first chemotherapy consultation, almost two years ago now, whether I had any questions. And I said, 'Yes, what do you do while you're having the treatment? You said it can take all day? Is it OK to watch DVDs?'

'Uh, sure,' Dr Ostler replied, looking a little quizzical, 'if you like. Though there aren't DVD players, I think there's just a regular TV in the room. But most people just chat to the nurse.' Huh, I remember thinking, not me. I'm not making conversation, I'm going to get as much distraction into that room as I can.

But the thing is, what seems fine in a hospital room – looking out for number one – is just too rude on home turf. You're in your living room, attached by see-through tubing to a plastic bag dripping liquid into your veins, a visit to the loo is out of the question, as is popping out to the kitchen to make a cup of tea. It's conversation or a particularly uncomfortable kind of silence. But both of us, Matt and I, seem more comfortable with some other activity to hand as well: so he sits with a clipboard on his lap making notes from time to time, and I marshal domestic tasks that don't involve too much concentration and mean I can make conversation at the same time.

But that, so far, is the only side effect of Herceptin I can record. Herceptin is a monoclonal antibody. It is pushed in through the veins, but it is a completely different experience from the chemotherapy drugs I had last year. I don't feel sick, I don't take cocktails of pills to counteract symptoms, it's just forty minutes or so on a drip.

So it isn't the clear, see-through drug that is keeping me from sleeping these nights. It's the fish. It starts the first night. We're out when they arrive and the children put them on the kitchen table with a note, 'From Angela (six exclamation marks); 4 Elon's birthday (eight exclamation marks and a smiley face).'

Something about them seems wrong as I head up to bed, and throughout the night I don't sleep. I keep going back downstairs then trudging up again to say, 'Anthony, I'm sure they're not supposed to be gasping for air like that – I think they're suffocating. Oh please, WAKE UP!'

It is the earliest moments of what will become an obsession. Three days later I'm at Maidenhead Aquatics – the local live-fish emporium – describing symptoms. 'You can't keep goldfish in something that size,' the guy is saying. His manner is laconic, like he's heard it all before, and he doesn't care that much anyhow. Not for the first time this year, I feel my age acutely. The last time I kept goldfish they lived in glass bowls about the size of a cabbage. And we think medicine's come a long way in the last twenty years. I return home from Maidenhead Aquatics with a hospital-room-sized fish tank, complete with fluorescent lighting, its own oxygen system and a planting scheme – apparently the minimum suitable accommodation for twenty-first-century goldfish.

None of it helps. Nearly halfway through my year's course of Herceptin, and Matt has tightened three holes on his belt, he informs me, but I can't keep three goldfish in good health in the most luxurious of conditions. And now, of course, Scott, the yellow one, the ugly one, has cancer. Or, at least, unexplained red bruising appearing through his skin, or scales, or whatever it's called.

It is a lesson for me – recorder of the ways of medical people – to be on the other side. I'm not the patient in this survival battle, but the one fighting to keep the bastards breathing. And it has completely filled my head, both waking and sleeping – I have a recurring goldfish dream these nights.

Not only has it driven into obscurity any concern with my own mortality, it's even given me a sense of perspective about the rejection letters in which I'm currently wading over my book proposal to write the story of these breast-cancer years – of which by far my favourite one so far, says: 'As you know, the breast-cancer memoir is a crowded market.' Finding myself yet again squatting, still as death, before the fish tank, trying to see whether Scott is, perhaps, just sleeping, I hear the words of the rejection letters playing through my head, and what I think is, 'Yes! Hurrah! Hallelujah for us. The breast-cancer memoir is a crowded market.' Because fish, you know, don't write.

People ask me all the time whether writing about the cancer is therapeutic. Or, instead of asking, they simply presume: 'It must be really helpful, having this outlet,' they say. Mostly, it's been a discipline, in the same way that having a very small child has kept me from spending days in bed. The response I get to the columns is often a practical bonus though – emails from all over the world, people writing from airports sometimes as they log on to the *Guardian*'s online editions. When I write in the news-paper about our fish, half a dozen people write and tell me the problem is overfeeding. Within days this proves to be true – though the fish-food packet instructs three times a day doses my correspondents tell me to feed the fish once, on alternate days only, and just a few flakes, six or seven. The red spots vanish within a week, and the green fug in the tank clears away.

I start to think again about my diet. Every so often over the past year I have tried to give up milk, which seems to be the most consistent piece of advice about diet and breast cancer. Or the bit that most applies to me, anyhow, since we already eat an organic-rich diet, with very little red meat, and as much fish as I can muster on to people's plates (less, now we have live ones in the house).

But my attempts have been half-heartedly successful at best, composed of internal arguments about how milk in coffee doesn't really count. All my doctors are adamant that there is no reason to give up milk, and that it is even a bad idea, because women are susceptible to osteoporosis.

While I was having radiotherapy I discussed it with Katherine Pigott, in charge of my treatment at the Royal Free Hospital. 'I did an Internet search,' she said. 'There is no basis at all for giving up milk. And,' she added, 'I have an adolescent daughter and I'm giving her full-fat milk, she has growing bones.' I stifled a sense of disquiet that the doctors are resorting to the Internet for their information and carried on drinking milk.

But when Elon's goldfish become so much healthier as soon as their diet is radically restricted I have another stab at giving up milk, pouring apple juice over cornflakes in the morning and grimacing. It doesn't work.

∽

These are the ways I know the cancer has come again. First, like Bridget Jones adding up alcohol units, there's a running total clicking through my head of how long each child is spending in front of various screens. I'm tired again. So when we come in from school, and Elon heads straight for the remote control, I just say, 'Yes, Cartoon Network, fine.' Then, sitting very still with tea in the kitchen, my brain is on a loop, making mad calculations: 'OK, children can have two hours TV/computer time a day before their minds frazzle, so if Elon watches two *Power Rangers* now, then I ask him to stop, that'll be OK, even if the big ones are watching *America's Next Top*

Model later on and he's in the room, because that's only another half an hour, and Nina's only been on MSN since four-thirty, and she goes to sleep around ten.'

Second, I find myself spurning hangers, trying to keep my touch light, seeking coloured clothes. 'I know there's a red tweed skirt in here,' I'm muttering, shuffling past the long black Nicole Farhi, the short black A-line cashmere from Camden Designers Market, the manifestations of black. Imperceptibly, as the chemotherapy, surgery and radiotherapy receded, and Herceptin became the once-in-three-weeks staple, I slipped once more into the easy uniform, the black on black. But it's back. I know this before I hear it from the consultant, I know it before I even make the appointment. I know it by the way I'm cruising my cupboard for colour, like some crazed garlic-warding quack. What did I do with that skirt?

Then the weight starts to drop off. For a year and a half I've been struggling to lose the steroid-induced stone, and suddenly I'm eating poppy-seed pastries with abandon, but dropping a pound a day. This is the real indictment of the times I have grown up in, more even than the fact that cancer is on the increase all around us. Cancer is running at one in three in the UK, one in four dying of it but, bad as that is, it seems to me worse that what really marks me as early-twenty-first-century woman is this: I'm welcoming the weight loss.

I have meetings with publishers these weeks. Suddenly, five have taken the bait, and I'm invited in to see all of them. I come back from the first one, with Simon and Schuster, and because I feel tired I make myself smoked mackerel on toast, but just looking at it makes me feel like throwing up, and I end up chucking it into the kitchen bin. 'Am I sick again?' I hear myself saying in my mind.

Last of all comes the fourth way, the scientific one. For as I note these symptoms in myself I start the inner calculations – do I call the doctors about this? First, there is some pain under my arm. One Friday night Anthony's mother says to me, gently, 'Dina, I have to tell you, you look so tired . . . is everything all right?'

I have been thinking for some days now whether or not I should go to see my doctors. But there is, always, a residual fear of seeming paranoid. The pain under my arm doesn't go away, though, so I phone Peter Ostler. I tell him about a meeting I have been invited to attend, with a group called the Cancer Campaigning Group, whose input is given to the government team that draws up five-yearly 'Cancer Plans'. And, while I'm talking to him, I say, 'Oh, and something else I should mention' as if it is incidental, and I tell him about the pain I've been feeling. There is only the slightest shading of concern in his voice, nothing to cause me any anxiety, just a raised alertness that tells me he is aware this is not small talk we are having.

'Yes,' he says, 'go and see Muhamed.' I don't tell Anthony or the kids that this appointment is anything other than routine, and Mr Al-Dubaisi, who looks grim when I come in, soon lightens considerably and says, after looking at my scar and feeling for lumps in all the usual places, 'There is nothing there.'

The next week, there is more good news. Thirteen

months after first taking my blood, the genetics screening team at Northwick Park, another North London hospital, tell me they can't find any mutation. The quiet geneticist apologizes wryly for the delay, saying if they could send the samples across the Atlantic to America they'd have the results in a fortnight, but their samples have to go across London to St George's Hospital, and 'St George's have a backlog'. If I'm not carrying a gene for breast cancer, that is good news for my daughters, of course. I phone Anthony to tell him, and he says, 'Well, what's caused it then?' The geneticist says, 'We don't know.'

I phone my parents also to spread these good results for my gene pool, but before I get the news out my mother says another first cousin has just come down with breast cancer – from which my grandmother died. I don't trust the genetic screen.

When two red blotches appear on the mastectomy scar I just note them, curse my dry skin, and double the doses of aqueous cream. The red patches are precise in shape, not really like the eczema I'm used to, and they don't itch. They also don't go away, no matter how much cream I use. I run over the symptoms Mr Al-Dubaisi mentioned: look out for backache, dyspepsia, but also, 'anything that doesn't go away'.

I register Anthony watching me check the marks in the mirror, but not saying anything. Fear of red marks. At my next Herceptin treatment, at home on the Jewish festival of Purim, Elon a red Power Ranger for the day, I take a quiet second with the nurse to say: 'Look, can I show you something, without worrying all this lot?' It is not Matt who has brought the medicine today, but another Healthcare at

Home nurse, a woman with a gentle manner. I'm glad –
I'm not sure I would have shown the marks to Matt.

I lift my shirt: 'Do you think it's anything?'

'Yes,' she says, 'I would get that checked.' I can't tell
from her voice if this is caution or serious. Her voice
seems blank of any intonation. So I ask her, when breast
cancer comes back, what does it look like? 'Usually,' she
says, 'usually it's a red rash.'

Fear. I practically have my shirt up almost before I'm
sitting opposite Mr Al-Dubaisi at the desk. 'I'm used to
this,' I gabble, apologizing for thrusting my chest at him.
He smiles, but his face has gone very still. He gestures to
the couch, calls in the nurse and draws the curtain
round.

'When did this come?' he says, troubled. 'You were
here just two weeks ago.' He is prodding the three spots
insistently, then springing his finger away again, as if he's
testing to see if the red stays.

Back at his desk, he has his palms together supporting
his chin in classic contemplative pose. 'What are you
thinking?' I say finally.

'I'm thinking when to do the biopsy,' he says. 'Is Friday
a religious day for you? What do you do on Friday?'

While he is thinking, he is also making calls. He tries
to get Peter Ostler on the phone, but only gets his message service. He goes through to Dr Ostler's colleague,
and asks some questions about Herceptin. When he gets
off the phone he looks at me, and says, 'I phoned him
because he knows more about Herceptin – I wanted to
find out if there was any chance you could get these kind
of red marks from taking the Herceptin. There isn't.'

In the end he does the biopsy that same night. I dial home, rearrange my teenagers, and Anthony comes to the Garden Clinic, the five-minute drive from our house. Mr Al-Dubaisi says he's giving me extra anaesthetic, 'so you have no pain at all'.

'Why isn't Dr Kaplan doing the biopsy?' I ask. First time round, Glenda Kaplan was in charge of biopsies; variations are making me anxious. I've been telling myself how I'll know my way round this time. Like how I'd be excellent at divorce a second time, having made every mistake possible first time. Although, I have to add, I never did get the wedding dress right, even second time.

Mr Al-Dubaisi looks at me quizzically. 'Why not Glenda?' I ask again.

'Because,' Mr Al-Dubaisi says, 'it's not in the breast. This is a surgeon's job, this biopsy, it's an excision of the skin.'

Of course, I don't have a breast there any more. And then, because this is the second time round, I persevere, heeding the mental voice saying, ask, if you don't understand. 'So is it skin cancer?' I say.

'No,' he answers. 'Skin cancer is a different type; there are many kinds of cancer. We don't know for sure until we do the tests, but yes, I believe I know what this is. It is a recurrence of the same breast cancer you had before, and it is in the chest wall.'

Mr Al-Dubaisi is the most cautious of speakers. For him to say anything definite, like 'I believe I know what this is', before he has the test results in front of him, is as good as a hundred test results. So when he says that, then I too know what it is.

Relationships become ragged as illness extends. Quite often these days Anthony says to me, 'Please tell me what you want; please don't assume I will know. I won't know, you have to tell me, but I do want to help.' I wasn't sure about phoning him to come along to this biopsy, not sure whether having him there would make it better or worse.

But when I am flat on my back on the raised white bed – 'I am not so tall,' Mr Al-Dubaisi always says to the nurses these days, 'can you make Dina higher?' – and packages of surgical implements wrapped in green cloths are being unwrapped and laid out on metal trolleys to my right, and Anthony is not flinching, but is lightly joking and calmly holding my hand, I am unspeakably glad he is there, and wonder how I ever go through any experiences without him.

After the biopsy Mr Al-Dubaisi asks if we have any more questions, but says, more or less, he can't answer anything until he has the test results. I am to come and see him after the weekend.

Back home, and one of our cats, Daisy, has wet Marganit's bed. I have this sense of everything crumbling, like the household is beginning to disintegrate with the return of the cancer. But one bed-change later and we're eating supper, Anthony, Marganit and I. Elon is in bed, Sara-Jenny is still out at her youth-group meeting, and Nina is on her way back from the latest of this year's Bat Mitzvah parties.

When she walks in she is trembling and her cheeks are red hot; she is running a fever. I sponge her down and tuck her into bed. Then Anthony and I slump on the couch to watch *The Apprentice*.

'Mum! Mum!' Nina is shrieking with pain from upstairs.

'Shhh, shhh, I'm here, what's wrong?' I say, straight into calm, nursing mode. But it isn't her temperature. She has heard her sisters whispering on the landing, about the cancer recurrence. 'It's OK,' I tell her. 'It's true, it is back, but it's going to be OK. You can see I'm all right, can't you?' I sit on her bed and stroke her arm.

We have guests on Friday night. Anything extra feels like an unbearable tension around my heart these days, an anxiety like in the early days of divorcing my first husband. Then, I remember having to force myself to carry on with the most mundane of tasks. Walking round the corner with a child in a buggy to buy bread, I would find my heart racing, I'd be trembling, and think I'd collapse, but because of the children this wasn't an option. I didn't even recognize it as divorce-induced anxiety, just understood I felt incredibly scared.

I have never had too little food on the table, but it remains a primeval source of fear that there will be people sitting expectantly around our table, and I won't have food to give them – my version of the 'walking naked down the street' nightmare. There are new sources of panic now, though, in between my Friday calculations of whether roast chicken, rice and salad is enough, or do we need asparagus, too? I do the 'anti-Ostler' and start checking websites. One of the first things Peter Ostler ever said to me was, 'Do be careful about going online – one or two websites, the NHS ones, are fine, but there's a lot of misinformation out there.'

After my initial diagnosis I took him at his word. Apart

from anything else I found so little time left over once the hurly-burly of treatments was factored into my ordinary work and home life, that I just didn't have time for long Internet browsing. Over the year and a half since those early days I'm aware of a slightly guilty sense that others are actively researching their treatments, and I'm not putting the necessary 'homework' into this disease.

So now I go online, typing the words 'breast cancer recurrence' into Google. One of the first things I read is, 'recurrence is about prolonging life, not about a cure'. The internal sensation these words produce feels like the old definition of cancer: something that eats away at the body from the inside. I feel that if I don't control it, don't stop it spreading, it will take me over and I'll disintegrate.

I am due to see Mr Al-Dubaisi Tuesday morning. By Monday lunchtime I have had enough of living in my head, and I phone Peter Ostler on his mobile, having tried Mr Al-Dubaisi's secretary first, only to get a recorded message saying she is on her annual leave.

I can hear in Dr Ostler's voice straight away that the news is not good. I say, 'Has Mr Al-Dubaisi spoken to you? Would you mind letting me know what the results of my biopsy are, if you have them?'

'Yes,' he says. 'I considered phoning you Friday night, actually, but . . .' This answers my question as to whether he even knows I've had a biopsy. 'It's not what we wanted to hear, I'm afraid,' he says. He sounds troubled.

'So is this connected to the pain I had under my arm?' I ask.

'Well, as you know, I got you to see Muhamed the same week you told me about the pain, and we didn't find anything.' I have the first intimations of a feeling that is going to recur; that I need to stifle any panic I feel at the notion that the doctors are now in the dark as much as I am.

I come off the phone, and go and see Anthony in his study down the corridor. He's stayed home from work today, a rare enough occurrence, partly because he has a sense of how I like to have a quiet daytime house in which to write. His staying home from work feels like a return to the first days of diagnosis, when he cancelled his office life for two weeks. I tell him what Peter Ostler has said. Tatiana and Milan are also in the house, and we all stand in the hall for a bit, shocked.

Later, I collect Sara-Jenny, Marganit and Nina from school and tell them too that it's confirmed the cancer has returned, but that it's probably local – 'the best kind of bad news'. I don't make a special point of sitting down with Elon to discuss it with him, because I don't think recurrence has any kind of meaning for him, but he hears when I talk to the other children, so I tell Elon, and also his teachers, that I will be having another hospital stay. I tell Elon there will be a magic cupboard again from which presents will spring forth, because I will be going to the same hospital.

The girls want to know if it will mean more chemotherapy, and I say I'm not sure. They seem to be taking it in their stride, but when we get home Nina bursts through the door and runs upstairs. She is on her bed, her body heaving with sobs. 'It will be OK,' I say to her. 'It will be OK.' I realize how they seem to think it's important they don't show me any grief, or any signs of perturbation at all, and I wonder how that has come about.

Thanks to my pre-emptive strike on Peter Ostler, Anthony and I already know the outline of what's happening to me before we go in to see Mr Al-Dubaisi the next morning. He looks grave, as he tells us it is a recurrence of the cancer, which of course we know already. It's local, he says, which means he can operate.

'I am confident it has not spread,' he says, hands together beneath his chin. It is unusual for him to be so open before he has any test results, and he is saying this before the scans and MRIs and blood tests. He is giving us all the reassurance in his power, even though it goes right against his medical instincts to speak before he has the proof. But, he explains, one can tell something about the nature of the cancer from the tissue taken in the biopsy, and so he can say that this does not seem to have spread to any organs.

He will operate, he says, and then perhaps there will be more radiotherapy. 'Because you are young, we will try everything,' he says, that rather discomfiting mantra the doctors use. Discomfiting, because what happens when I'm sitting before them with a recurrence aged seventy?

'I need to excise the area,' he says. I ask him what he means, and he starts to explain about a bone scan, which will confirm the cancer has not spread.

'No, no,' I say, 'what does excise mean?'

He says, 'Oh, that means I will cut out the tumours,' and with his hands he sketches a long oval shape.

'So what's involved in this surgery?' I ask, but he is not ready for a long discussion about this yet.

'Well, first I must examine you again, and then we will discuss it further.'

Sister Briodie, the breast-care nurse, is already in position next to my assigned place on the couch behind the curtain. She busies herself tidying up discarded clothes, calling in the surgeon when I am undressed and lying down.

He looks at the area and shows me on my body the bits he will cut out. He says the scar will be vertical, going upwards from the present one which is horizontal. 'I'm happy to operate,' he says, very brisk. I have the sense that I only ever get the shadiest glimpse of the calculations he makes in his mind about each surgery.

Back at his desk, he is in expansive mode again. He says mine was always a 'Grade Three tumour, with lymph node and vascular involvement'. I have only the vaguest understanding of these terms, combined with a feeling that this is the sort of thing other patients inform themselves about. In essence, he says, the kind of tumour I had was always likely to return; Herceptin gives a 50 per cent less likelihood of return, but mine may have been given too late, more than six months after finishing chemotherapy. It should be given straight after the chemotherapy, Mr Al-Dubaisi says. This is something that becomes a low-level point of discussion over the next months. I put the point to Peter Ostler: was the Herceptin given in time or not? He tells me it was.

There is the first laughter in the room when Mr Al-Dubaisi phones Dr Ostler to book one of the scans, and Ostler apparently says he's already spoken to me and confirmed the diagnosis. 'She didn't tell me that,' Mr

Al-Dubaisi comments with a smile. 'She's sitting right here in front of me.'

We discuss the old question of the second opinion, and as quickly reject it. The time it would take to make an appointment and see somebody else would delay the surgery, so, having toyed with the idea, we – Anthony and I – have already rejected it. And that's what I say to Mr Al-Dubaisi: 'There's no point, really, is there? It's not like you're saying there's one possible treatment, and then there's also this other one, and we have a choice to make. Really, this is just a question of surgery.' He nods.

So sure am I of this man and his reluctance to say a word too early, that I go home and tell the children: 'It has not spread, Mr Al-Dubaisi says so. And Mr Al-Dubaisi is a man who would not say it is raining, even if rain was pouring against the windows, unless he himself was outside feeling rain, and testing it with his surgeon's hands'.

That night it's mega-selling children's author Anthony Horowitz's latest book launch, at the residence of the Ambassador from Peru, a bemused-looking man with a very courteous manner.

There are children's book launches most weeks, most nights of the week some parts of the year, but though I pile up the invitations in the kitchen I rarely manage to attend, because the early evening start times of these bright-lights dos coincide exactly with the timing of my home-based children's book activities: in the dim glow next to Elon's bed, reading just one more story.

But tonight I force myself out, a Scott Fitzgerald heroine in search of therapy. Also, Anthony Horowitz is one of the authors I feel I know a bit – I've interviewed him twice, and he came to Hasmonean High School, the school I attended and where Sara-Jenny, Marganit and Nina now go, to speak to the children in assembly.

I first interviewed him in June 2003 when, I suppose, he was just becoming the household name he is now. Most adults know the names of only one or two of the children's authors: J. K. Rowling, of course, and then possibly Philip Pullman and Jacqueline Wilson. But all the children know Anthony Horowitz and his boy hero, Alex Rider. The children have been faster than the grown-ups to identify the hot names in children's publishing, which is flourishing this early part of the century.

I remember a Saturday lunch at our house some years back, 2000, I think, just us, the kids and one of England's top books editors with his wife. His wife, talking to my eleven-year-old, mentioned she had a review copy of the newest *Harry Potter*. Electric excitement around the table. The only ones who looked puzzled, and said, 'Who? What?' were the editor, and my Anthony – no mean literary critic himself. This wasn't the first Harry Potter – it was the third.

In our house, though, Horowitz has not been overlooked by grown-ups. Fantastically prolific, he has a separate string to his bow, writing television scripts. His series, *Foyle's War*, gentle Second World War detective stories in sleepy English backwaters, is my husband's viewing of choice, and quite often playing in the background on the laptop while Anthony is simultaneously working on his desktop.

Horowitz has something of the adolescent boy about

him, like a lot of the children's authors who keep their 'inner child'. At the party this night he is radiating good health but also pride – his own teenage sons are in attendance, tall, dark and good-looking like the heroes of his books, and Horowitz is beaming.

In a corner of the room some of us are talking, about tonsil operations and burglaries and bad stuff that's been happening. Maybe because I'm tired, when somebody says, 'Anyhow, you're looking really well, Dina, that's great,' I actually tell them.

I say, 'Oh, in fact, it's come back, my tumour. They're operating on Tuesday. Turns out it's not such a brave new Herceptin world, after all.'

The group I'm standing in goes awkward. Faces register concern, but spiked with discomfort, and bodies shift. And I realize that what I've said is the literal truth. It's not such a brave new world, and cancer's not just a sickness, it remains a taboo. Back home I write about the party in the latest of the notebooks I've been keeping ever since the breast cancer started.

I have failed to write every day in this, the sixth of these notebooks, as regular life overtook breast cancer. I turn back to the first page which starts with my Herceptin treatments, but then carries on mostly with details of Theo's Bar Mitzvah, Nina's Bat Mitzvah, Elon starting school in earnest, Sara-Jenny in her last year of secondary school, me wondering – yet again – what to wear: what do I wear to go on morning television to talk about children's books? Will there be new embarrassments, previously unimagined, because of having a microphone tucked down my single-breasted front? What to wear to evening dos? What to wear when it's hot?

One day a stylist called Gok comes to the house to prepare me for a magazine piece about post-mastectomy clothes. He's young, nice and dressed in black leathers and a white shirt. 'I understand exactly how you feel,' he says to me, 'to me it's everything, how I look when I walk out on the street.' Then he opens my cupboard to see what material we have to work with. 'Uh,' he says, turning back in some dismay to the magazine's features editor sitting perched on my bed, 'I think we'll call some stuff in.'

A bit later, he turns to me, a little puzzled, and says, 'Why don't you want to put on a prosthesis?' I explain, yet again, how it feels humiliating to be stuffing fake cloth down one side of a bra, but also how even the softest mastectomy bra is not comfortable over the scarred area. I wear thin cotton singlets every day as a first layer.

Many times in this sixth notebook I have written: 'life getting back to normal, really need to sort my working routines out again'.

Tonight I scribble a closing line on the final page of the book I'd labelled 'Home Run' – decorating it with lots of exclamation marks and stars to make it suitably celebratory, a farewell to breast cancer: 'Huh, guess this won't be last notebook after all.'

16. Because You are Young, Dina

The series of tests are already booked before we leave Mr Al-Dubaisi's office. The CT scan is first, in a mobile unit that drives around the country and has landed in this corner of North London, a hospital called 'BUPA Bushey', in time for me. I wake up at five to eat some cereal. You mustn't have any food for four hours before the CT scan, and breakfast is my favourite meal. Last night Anthony drove round the late-night supermarkets culling different cereals to bring home to me. Marganit has left a new copy of *Harpers and Queen* magazine on the kitchen table.

After dropping Elon at school, Anthony and I drive off to Bushey. I have to finish four cups of some white frothing liquid before the scan. As if this isn't bad enough the receptionists are busily detailing their respective Botox treatments. One of them swears by a primer, whose name I never catch. The other secretary finally leaves, to take her daughter for hair extensions.

Finally it's time for me to go out to the scanner, which is in a large grey and white Portakabin. The nurse says Anthony will have to wait inside the main building. So I climb the six iron steps and inside I change into one of the usual back-opening gowns. I don't understand why hospital gowns are back-opening, but I do know it is something that makes me feel more vulnerable, more exposed.

To do this scan, the doctors shoot iodine round your veins, through a needle. Only the iodine bursts right through my veins, an explosion that gets everybody running, while at the same time saying, 'This is absolutely fine, no problem, you'll get a big bruise though.' Actually, apart from a few seconds, they're right, it doesn't hurt. It looks bad, though; my left arm instantly grows huge mounds, like Popeye muscles.

The doctor has another stab. I say to the two nurses, 'Can you please call my husband in?' The blonde one, the English nurse, nods and says yes. A minute later I can see they are all still in the mobile unit with me: the English doctor, the English nurse, and the black-haired nurse from Australia.

'If you are all in here, who is calling Anthony?' I say.

'We usually keep people out of the scanning area,' one of them mutters.

'You're nowhere near scanning yet,' I say. 'You're just trying to put the needle in. I would like Anthony in here, please.'

I have to ask three more times. Later Anthony tells me the nurse came out and said, 'Can you come and calm your wife down please; she's becoming overemotional.'

They never do get that needle in, and we leave in a flurry of insincere-sounding 'anything else you want to know, Dina?' and 'you'll have a huge bruise' comments. An hour later I am in the front hall of Elon's school collaring parents as they arrive to collect their children; we need to rustle up some support for sales of the school calendar, a new project, featuring pictures of the children and, for five pounds to the parent teacher association, each child's birthday listed on its day in the calendar. I stand in the doorway, my Popeye-d arm concealed beneath a baggy jacket, and don't let anybody past until they pledge their money.

Next day, in London's Wimpole Street, at the London Imaging Centre, I meet 'it'. The doctor who can both do his medical stuff and has the bedside manner to go with it.

Ian Renfrew is called by the radiologist – the same woman who, so many months ago, first breezily injected me when I was initially diagnosed and Mr Al-Dubaisi wanted to find out whether or not the cancer had spread – to look at my arm. The first time I met her she was completely confident about her ability to inject. 'Don't worry,' she had said to me, smiling when she saw me tense, 'I have many years of doing this.' But today she takes one look and says she will call somebody else; she doesn't want to try putting a needle into a bruised limb.

Dr Renfrew strides in, checked shirt under forest-green jumper with pink edging, and mutters, 'Shocking.'

'Really?' I say. 'Really? Is it shocking? Because whenever they can't get needles in, they say that it's my veins which are no good.'

'Where is Bushey, anyhow?' Dr Renfrew asks me. 'I was at medical school with a guy from Bushey, never knew where it was, but he ended up as a jingle on the radio: I'm Ba-aa-a-a-rry from Bushey . . .' The needle is in, and the bone and CT scan completed almost before the smile has left my face. He even says I don't need to drink the bubbling white liquid, the barium drink that tastes like milk of magnesia: 'The truth is it's not necessary: unless you're stupid you can tell a lymph node from a bowel.'

The gowns here are also back-opening, but you are given a soft white dressing gown to wear over it, which feels so much less exposing. The CT scan is a strange sensation, like your body being flooded with hot liquid. 'You'll feel like you need to pee,' the scan operator says, 'but don't worry, you won't.'

By the end of the week I am back in the Garden Hospital for Mr Al-Dubaisi's second attempt at removing the cancer. Once again the tests have shown the cancer is local, and he says, very firmly, that he will remove it.

And so to hospital, equipped with a 'smooshie' – a foam-filled blue fish-shaped cushion – from my children, which lodges so perfectly around my neck on hospital pillows it becomes something of an obsession with me, a copy of *Julie and Julia*, by Julie Powell, and *Beware of God* by Shalom Auslander, one of the best books I've ever read, I think, and when I sleep I keep it close to my head, revelling in its understanding of Jewish life, which is as complete as its irreverence for that life.

Anthony and Sara-Jenny walk me to the lift to head down to the operating theatre, and I'm already looking forward to the excellent and deep sleep provided by anaesthetic. I crave deep sleep, and am perfectly happy to smile sweetly at the anaesthetist's usual jokes about 'off to the Maldives, first class' en route to oblivion.

I wake up, too soon, in recovery, not back in the bedroom yet, to hear Mr Al-Dubaisi saying, 'Dina, Dina.' I think he is trying to bring me back to consciousness. 'She gave me a hard time,' I think I hear him say, then he is standing over me, saying kindly, 'That's all right, now.'

I ask what the time is and remember thinking I should ask about Elon, while realizing at the same time that it's OK, I don't have to worry about Elon, because I'm in hospital and somebody else is in charge of my life right now.

Two days later I'm back home and cross with myself for shouting at the girls to tidy up their bedrooms. Somehow, Pesach – Passover – is looming once again, my hospital week has been preceded by half a dozen publishers' meetings but nobody is offering very much money for my book, Marganit is up too late each night finishing coursework for her GCSE exams, Sara-Jenny needs to sort out her driving test, and Anthony is deep in assorted debates about whether the Left in this country is fostering anti-Semitism.

The clenching fear about the cancer lodges somewhere beneath.

Mr Al-Dubaisi debriefs us. Either because his English is not perfect, or because my situation is not that clear any more, neither Anthony nor I leave the meeting feeling as if we understand what the future holds. Mr Al-Dubaisi says the report on the tumour he removed shows that 'we got everything out, but there is lymph activity at one centimetre'. He is concerned about this, he tells us, so he discussed with two senior colleagues – and his slightly vulnerable expression reveals the difficult territory we are in – whether to operate again, but all have agreed this would not be a good idea. Also, I can't have any more radiotherapy because I have already been given the highest dose possible.

I feel myself tuning out of the conversation, as I often do, while Anthony and Mr Al-Dubaisi debate my health. 'I am a litigator,' Anthony says, 'so I look for the worst scenarios.'

'You are right and sensible to do that, Anthony,' the surgeon replies.

I feel sick and worried, and in my mind I am thinking, no way am I dying until Elon is in his twenties. Make that thirties, I tell myself. Then Sara-Jenny will be in her forties, which is where I am now, and that's OK. I am deep into these internal calculations as Mr Al-Dubaisi checks the new scar where my right breast used to be. 'It is healing nicely,' he says, and I cannot match those words with the actual sensation of this stitched area of my body, which feels dry, hard, like grating.

Back home there is an email from *Jewish Book Week*, responding to a piece of mine that's just appeared in the *Jewish Chronicle*, about going to the mikvah, the ritual baths in which observant women immerse themselves following their periods, after mastectomy.

It is like this in the mikvah, always. A moment of complete awareness of self. It comes from the oddness of being about to embark on the most private of rituals in surroundings that aren't your own.

It happens just after you walk in to the individual bathroom, when the sometimes over-fussy, sometimes gently discreet mikvah attendant has left you alone with the towels, and the packs of cotton buds, and the emery boards, and you're absorbing the slight strangeness of being alone, in a room which still bears the faint breath of the woman who came before. It's the mix of intimacy and alien-ness that heightens your awareness like that, in the quiet of those bathrooms, decorated in their invariable pastel shades.

But these days it's not the way it ever was for me before. Because I am post-mastectomy. Not once, not ever, did I imagine being single-breasted in the mikvah. I thought I'd come to terms with the operation, happy to walk around as casually at home as ever I did.

Sitting here, on the edge of the bath, I suddenly realize I'm not sure I'm ready to see a relative stranger's reaction to my operated-on body. Why? I keep asking myself. You've had two years under a barrage of medical treatments, lying like a fish on a slab having radiotherapy; three-weekly appointments with a needle up my arm, and the thorough checks by doctors I've only just met. Surely I'm beyond feeling tense in front of strangers.

What's different about the mikvah? Well, there's the rush of emotions it induces. The sense of having come to terms with having been menopaused by medical science, only to find that hasn't happened after all. It's that extraordinary way Judaism does this full-frontal dealing with sex, making it so blatant a big deal that you go through a whole ceremony marking it out, making you confront the wear and tear of life, the shifting patterns. And for cancer patients, like me, I think one of the most frightening things of all is the physical self scrutiny involved in the mikvah rituals.

The post-treatment period is a lonely time for cancer patients: scared to be a nuisance to over-stretched doctors, wondering if you have just become too conscious of ordinary physical changes. In the mikvah, it's part of the process, minutely checking every part of yourself before you walk down those steps into the water. Carrying cancer and suddenly every raised bump, every reddish patch raises the question: is it back?

The email from the director of *Jewish Book Week* asks if I will launch my book at their annual event. I don't even have a publisher yet! But Tracy, my agent, says I should accept the offer from Simon and Schuster. So now, within days of my second operation to remove cancer, I have a launch event and a publisher.

17. Metastasis

Seventy-five thousand and eighty-five pounds, and fourteen pence. One month after my second operation – three more bits of cancer surgically excised from my body – and I'm doing a very un-British thing at my kitchen table. I'm adding up the cost of my treatment to date, while Matt dispenses intravenous Herceptin.

The £75, 085.14 running total is, coincidentally, exactly ten times (less the eighty-five pounds and fourteen pence) the advance royalty I'm receiving for my book about having breast cancer. So, my life is worth ten times more than my thoughts on my life. Chasteningly, that is a gap that is getting ever wider; the royalty is fixed but I'm still having treatments, and/or diagnostic scans of one sort or another most weeks.

Though I've lived in London on and off since I was nine, I was born in Charleston, South Carolina, and I can tell it's my American roots showing today because of the look on Matt's face, which is just slightly wide-eyed at what I am doing in public, so to speak. Still, he's concentrating on the job, finding a vein running up my arm that will take the needle, which is an increasingly tense business as the months and months of intravenous treatment go by.

Normally, it's an anxious moment for both of us, attempting light chat so as to take my mind off the matter in, quite literally, my hand. But today, while Matt, a ruddy fellow, is white with the effort of not jabbing me too often before hitting a vein that will work, I am concentrating elsewhere. It's engrossing finding out how much things cost, and during this Herceptin dose is a perfect time to be doing it.

Increasingly, I need ever harder-core diversions to distract from what's happening to my body; for example, while Mr Al-Dubaisi snips out the stitches from what used to be my right breast, I lie back and muse about how these doctors are when they confront their partners' breasts in bed. Money is hard-core in British society. I know this because I am always asking the children's authors I interview what their advance and royalty deals are: Americans tell me as readily as the British look horrified by the question. (With, in three years of covering them, just one exception: Frank Cottrell Boyce, a writer from Liverpool who pens fast-paced children's novels, *Framed* and *Millions*. He readily told me about his earnings: '£150,000 for the first two books, then £250,000 for the forthcoming two.' A hit screenwriter – *Jackie and Hilary*, *Cock and Bull Story*, just two of his credits – he said he often made no money from movies at all. Although, comically, when I publish that quote from Frank in the *Guardian*, he emails me the next day to say he was actually visiting a friend with cancer, and had brought the usual small gift that one might take to somebody ill, only to have the newspaper brandished in his face and ending up having to buy the whole neighbourhood chicken takeaways that night.)

Ever since being diagnosed with this illness I've kept a flimsy yellow paper folder stuffed into the bookshelf next to my desk. Each time one of the insurance slips comes through, with the printed words 'payments direct to the hospital or specialist' (in bold) and the actual amounts (in normal font) listed beneath, I chuck the slip in the folder. The yellow folder, which seemed perfectly fine for the job when this all began, is of course fit to burst by now, like a Texan on fast food. Today, I'm adding all the amounts, out loud of course, because I had an English state school maths education, and so understand numbers simply as slippery things that need firm handling: two calculators and very clear enunciation of the amounts as I go. From Matt's air I'd say he finds the proceedings both interesting and mildly transgressive.

'Huh, Dr Ostler, £380 every time he opens his mouth (and worth it, and worth it, I mutter in Matt's direction); £3165.48, so that's what a mastectomy costs these days, which bit's the forty-eight pence do you suppose? Ah yes, here come the £2018 amounts, that's the Taxotere, and oh yes, wow, here we go, this must be you chaps, Healthcare at Home, uh, £3019.88, hmm.' To all of which Matt listens with what I consider to be a particularly English expression on his face, composed of one-ear cocked in beady interest combined with a slight manner of humouring naughty children in the nursery.

He resolves this inner conflict by joining in full-frontally: 'The odd pennies are the VAT (value added tax) amounts added in,' he explains. And, 'doctors have to pay for their licences, very expensive, more than us nurses'.

This is due to be one of my last Herceptin treatments. The question is, what's next? Do I just sit around and wait for the cancer to rear again, or do the doctors have any tricks left?

That's the long-term discussion anyhow. The short-term one is rather more urgent: will my skin ever heal from this second bout of surgery, or am I going to need a skin graft? So far it's not looking good. Because Mr Al-Dubaisi had to operate on the area where I had a mastectomy, and because that area was treated by radio-therapy, the skin there is already damaged from radiation and therefore less inclined to heal.

The first time they try to remove the stitches the entire wound pops open again, and the gentle nurse is soon set-ting up a mini-operating table for Mr Al-Dubaisi to restitch the area. Always ready with the obvious question I ask, 'Uh, is this going to hurt?'

'No, no,' Mr Al-Dubaisi says, 'I will give you a local anaesthetic. The only bit which will hurt will be that needle giving the local.'

'I'm absolutely happy to have a general anaesthetic,' I say. Everybody seems busy, and nobody answers, so I repeat it.

'I don't think we have time for that,' Mr Al-Dubaisi says.

Then he washes the area out with iodine, and I am screeching in pain. He looks almost as unhappy as I feel, but says quietly he has to make sure the area is disinfec-ted, that's his main concern. He dilutes the iodine with water, though, which is better.

When it comes to doing the stitching, he says with

some feeling, 'Dina, can you please turn your head the other way?' and I realize it's not just hard on the patient when procedures have to be done under local rather than general anaesthetic.

The stitches have already been in for thirteen days but he decides he'll leave them in for several more weeks. I'm assuming I will need a skin graft because a friend in the same situation said that's what happened to her, but that, it turns out, is to underestimate the determination and skill of Mr Al-Dubaisi.

He gives me a couple of weeks to 'rest and relax' – two weeks which coincide with Pesach and the children's spring holiday from school, not to mention firming up the plans for Nina's Bat Mitzvah, which involves trans-porting sixty children and food to an indoor snow-slope for an afternoon's skiing and snow-boarding, and, at the back of my mind, making early plans for Anthony's immi-nent fiftieth birthday.

It is exactly six weeks and two days since the operation when I meet up with Mr Al-Dubaisi again for his next attempt at removing the stitches. The simple procedure is surprisingly upsetting. It feels like there is a zipper grown suddenly on my body, and the skin is so rough. The sur-geon has to tug with some strength to remove the stitches, and the nurse who is assisting him, whose name accord-ing to her badge is 'Feely', says: 'Hmm, that looks like hard work.'

At some level, right near the surface in fact, I don't really believe that this has happened to me. When I do feel the sorrow, my immediate reaction is to stifle it, stem the source, not let it overwhelm.

I concentrate on Mr Al-Dubaisi's impeccable courtesies: the way he pulls over a towel to cover my left breast while he works on the right side, with an impatient shrug because the nurse hasn't bothered to do this already; his efforts to engage me in small talk, which doesn't come easily to him, because he is anxious to distract me from what is happening. When the last stitch is removed, minute pieces of what looks like fine blue nylon, the sort they use in fishing reels, the surgeon allows himself the smallest sigh of relief. To me, he simply says, 'Yes, that is fine now, that will not reopen.'

I ask him, chirpily, about reconstruction, the bulky term the doctors use for the operation that gives you back a breast. He doesn't miss a beat, replying, 'Not for a year at least.'

After, at his desk, we talk again about further radiotherapy, an option already mooted, but then rejected because I've had the maximum radiation dose to the area and if I have any more the skin will go 'necrotic' – basically it will die. He repeats this, saying he has discussed the question with several people. He says my cancer was always an 'aggressive' type, and that there is some evidence of lymph node activity. I don't really take in what he is saying, and am confused by the talk about the operation having been successful – the cancer removed – followed by the negative news about lymph node 'activity'.

Maybe it's the effect of having the stitches removed – nothing holding me together any more – or maybe it's just cancer the second time round, but I feel like I need a bracing dose of iodine swilling round my thought processes. I feel more panicky than before and also more susceptible to the people who write to me, telling me to change my diet, change my mind-set. It leads to sleepless nights. I'd like to wash away all the conflicting information.

I find myself obsessively checking the Nottingham Prognostic Index, a calculating tool you can read on the Internet, by which you multiply the grade of your tumour by 0.2 and add the stage of your cancer, or some such formula of little meaning to the mathematically challenged amongst us, and then you can find out whether your chemotherapy is going to work or not. Or something.

I say to Peter Ostler two completely opposing things. First, 'What is the point of my carrying on with the Herceptin? Obviously it hasn't worked.'

'No, you've got that wrong,' he says, annoyed initially, but quickly correcting and moderating his tone. 'To us,' he says, 'the good thing is that your cancer hasn't spread. It's remained local.' I stare at him, bleary-eyed, tired from my nights up with a calculator and the NPI, attempting to take control of my treatment, as all the best people writing to me courtesy of my *Guardian* column tell me to do.

So then I say, 'So why stop at eighteen doses? Why don't I take it for two years, or three years? Or forever?' I ask.

'The evidence base isn't there,' he says.

∽

Do you feel all right? This is the question the doctors ask me every time they see me now, and I seem to have appointments most weeks. 'We will be keeping a close eye on Dina,' are the words Mr Al-Dubaisi uses to Anthony.

'I don't know,' I say, mulish, when asked about my welfare by medical staff. 'You tell me how I am.' My instincts are necrotized, I want independent confirmation of everything.

'Look, any problems at all, don't feel you are bothering us,' both Dr Ostler and Mr Al-Dubaisi say, repeatedly, 'just come for a check-up.'

In fact, the reassurance I'm after is daily scans; no sooner does that cross my mind than I simultaneously dismiss it as a ridiculous request, of course, no way can I ask for that, I don't even tell anybody that's what I'm thinking. Anthony, though, successful in this town and privately educated – and so with a completely different sense of what's owing to him – puts the very question. 'Surely Dina should be scanned every week,' he says to Mr Al-Dubaisi one time when I am not in the room.

'To find out what?' Mr Al-Dubaisi says.

'Whether the cancer has spread,' my husband answers.

'What is the point of knowing that?' the surgeon replies. In a middle-eastern way that I recognize, Mr Al-Dubaisi is saying, let us deal with that when that time comes, let us not run to meet it.

All my life, as a journalist, I've resisted the notion that there are any questions at all that are better left unanswered, or indeed unasked. My report cards from school were replete with phrases like, 'Dina asks too many questions. She is attention-seeking, and a distraction to her fellow students.' But now I find myself policing my own mind, telling myself to stop asking stuff. My mind, at least, I can aspire to controlling.

Other people remain unpredictable though. A very young-sounding girl from the Arts desk at the *Guardian* telephones one quiet morning. 'Hope this doesn't sound too callous, but there's this new French film about a thirty-one-year-old man dying of cancer; we wondered if you'd mind going to see it for us, and writing a couple of hundred words about whether it seems realistic or not?'

I laugh and negotiate the fee up a hundred pounds, making it the most the *Guardian* has ever paid for a commission of just a couple of paragraphs. Later, telling a friend about the call, I say, 'and can you believe this? I heard myself saying to her, "Thank you for thinking of me"!'

But there is something bracing about having journalistic calls on my life during this period thrust back into the tunnel of cancer treatment. In the circumspect and lowered-speech world of this illness, treated by doctors and nurses whose voices audibly change register as they shift from talking to colleagues to talking – ever so slightly kinder and more slowly – to you, the patient, it has been, quite simply, just great to be talking from time to time with journalists.

When the columns first started running, my editor, Ian, phoned late one afternoon to say, 'I don't think we can have quite so much about breasts next week, Dina. Don't forget you have to keep readers like me too.'

And it is Ian who puts to me quite directly a question I can see in other people's eyes. 'So,' he says, with a quizzical, lopsided smile, 'have you asked . . . you know . . . how many years?'

Just over two months from the second operation to remove the cancer, after many nights of waking up trembling from dreams about Grade Three tumours, Stage Three cancers – conscious while I'm dreaming that I am still not entirely clear what those terms mean – Ian's question becomes the only question in the room.

It is on my birthday – no surprise – a sunny, warm Friday, at five in the afternoon, the hospital waiting room cleared, the week's urgencies sorted, the dozy weekend settling over the wards like a mushroom cloud – that Peter Ostler calls Anthony and me back into his office, and he has a colleague with him.

I know what the presence of 'the colleague' means as loud and clear as if he was wearing a black-edged placard round his neck saying, 'Death Row'. I can't even look at the colleague while the doctors speak to us. I look at Peter Ostler, and I know in my eyes there's an expression of complete betrayal: how could you let this happen to me, I put my trust in you? I do not think Dr Ostler could look more upset, but I am unrelenting. When his colleague, David Mills, speaks, I look away, look out of the window, hum underneath my breath like a recalcitrant schoolgirl, metaphorically sitting there with fingers stuck in my ears, refusing to listen. Because he is the symbol of the bad news. There has never been the need for 'a colleague' in the room before.

They are not good at giving this news, the news of metastasis, the spreading of the cancer – as bad as I am at receiving it in fact. They say, 'Well, it is what we feared.

It's no longer local, there are signs of lymph nodes in the abdomen and the chest wall.'

But while they discuss options they also joke with each other, trying to ease the tension, segueing into a double act, about how one has been to Florida while 'the other stayed here doing all the work'. Anthony, lawyer, literary critic, husband, can't get over this. Later, he keeps on repeating it, his shock at what he calls their autism, their way of dealing with us. 'Do they think we care about their work trips?' he says.

And he is the one who is surprised that Mr Al-Dubaisi never phones. He mentions it to Peter Ostler the following week. 'I would have thought the surgeon would phone us,' he says. Dr Ostler shrugs his shoulders, says these are always difficult decisions, knowing how to manage these times for patients, but it's not a sign of lack of concern.

∞

It is the morning that coincides with my eighteenth dose of herceptin that the red blotches came back again. 'I think if it was cancer, the marks would be more red,' says today's nurse, a woman who chats away about organizing her young daughters so one can go to Brownies while the other does homework.

But I phone Mr Al-Dubaisi's secretary anyhow. 'Could you just let him know I think the cancer's back?' I say, as baldly as that. The anxiety is intense. I feel nauseous and short of breath – am I imagining these symptoms? The coughing and the sense of not being able to breathe is new.

I know as soon as I see Mr Al-Dubaisi's face that the cancer has, indeed, reappeared, its third manifestation. No biopsy required this time to test it out. He just has to look. 'I am happy to operate again,' he says confidently. We fill the silence in the room with banter. He spots an enraged-looking mosquito bite on my arm, and immediately writes out a prescription for antibiotics.

'Wow,' I say to Anthony, 'I really am a top-gun patient now: antibiotics for a mosquito bite!'

Mr Al-Dubaisi smiles gently. 'We need to watch that bite, you need to make sure you don't catch infections.'

'Are you going to surgically remove my mosquito bites too from now on?' I joke as we leave the room.

When we go back home I tell the children, and they say, 'Isn't that a bit soon?' It never crosses my mind not to tell the children, though everybody is in the throes of end-of-year tests and final exams and driving tests. There is no screaming or crying any more when they hear this kind of news; I don't see them talking in whispers. But their anxiety shows over the next few days when they text regularly – have you had your scan yet?

The scans are the staging process, as I now know it is called. The CT, the MRI, the bone scan – the machines that say the cancer is local (and curable) or that it has spread. The hospital scanner breaks down so the CT scan to check where the cancer is gets delayed.

And so it should have been Thursday we heard the bad news, but of course it's the Friday, my birthday. My girls are at their father for the weekend, we have Anthony's children, his mother and a family friend for dinner in a couple of hours. We're driving home, and I'm saying to myself, think calmly, think what's best for the children – don't get fixated on your promise to them to tell them what's going on as soon as it happens.

I break the promise. I don't tell the girls as soon as I hear the news myself. I say to Anthony, let's not disrupt the contact arrangements for this; it makes it all too urgent. Let's not tell anybody for a few days – just us. 'Like during the divorces,' he says, 'just each other to rely on.'

When Anthony and I were going through our respective tortured divorces, we had a daily mantra, which went like this: 'Just imagine the worst thing possible happening, and it will happen.' It was a way of facing down trouble, not being taken by surprise.

Like a microcosm of the battle between parenting gurus over the last century, we have these different parenting styles, Anthony and me. He doesn't do 'parenting' with a capital P, and hasn't – I don't think – looked at a parenting book in his life. I've read them all, and have absorbed intravenously the notion that consistency is incredibly important to children. They can come through anything if they know you will always tell them the truth, and your ground won't shift.

But actually, it's good, breaking my rule on this occasion – the promise to tell them everything as soon as it happens. Because Friday night feels like the end of my life, but by the next morning I feel lighter. I look in the mirror, and I don't see a dying person. I think the doctors gave us the news in too desperate a way, their brows too gloomy, their eyelids too hooded.

I have symptoms, sure. I feel nauseous – again, like

pregnancy, so I can't face making meals. I fantasize about perfectly balanced, easily digestible meals appearing without any shopping or planning required from me at all. I sort this out by subscribing to the *Guardian*'s 'eat-right' plan, a nutrition programme I can access online. This is a canny move. Each week my computer offers up a week's list of menus and a shopping list, which I order from an online supermarket straight away. I think the change to our suppers is so remarkable everybody will comment.

I notice the children eating up. But nobody says a word. It's exactly three weeks and two days before one daughter says, 'I really like this food you're making, what is this?' (Marinated Quorn, as it happens, that night.) The 'eat-right' missives work on so many levels. I feel I need to eat to keep strong, and the meal plans trick the nausea by constantly varying the ingredients. I could not, these days, stomach making, or swallowing, my ideal healthy meal of fish and green vegetables every night. These 'eat-right' meals come with panoplies of ingredients that change frequently, faster than my mind can register 'ugh, I can't eat that'. So I'm cooking food for multi-examined students, somebody else is doing the thinking for me; it's great.

And while this is going on, Anthony and I are hitting the telephones. One of his clients is a major breast-cancer research benefactor, and one morning Anthony, with the restlessness of an active man used to finding solutions to problems, asks his client for names: the best in the business, who they are and their direct lines.

Two years to the day since my first diagnosis, we do,

finally, call in the second opinions. We speak to doctors at Johns Hopkins, at Sloan Kettering, at Tulane and in Paris; doctors who phone me from their mobiles with information and comforting messages. 'Don't be frightened,' they say, 'there are many options.' This is a crucial phrase, and it's not one my doctors used. It's a difference in style.

We also, on Peter Ostler's recommendation, go to see a doctor in the UK, Stephen Johnston at the Royal Marsden. His office is more luxurious than the curtained-off bit of hallway where Dr Ostler has to see patients at Mount Vernon, and this makes a difference, gives the consultation a feel of stability rather than panic.

Professor Johnston has a screen, which, at the touch of a button, lights up so he can display my x-rays and make points like a lecturer. He explains why the Herceptin may have failed me, saying that sometimes the Her-2 protein doesn't recognize Herceptin, and also that doctors are realizing that a combination of drugs, mixing Herceptin with some other agent, is sometimes necessary. He also tells us that now they know it is not just Her-2 which is involved, but other bits of the protein being produced by the tumour, called Her-1, 3 and 4.

He also says, in that same calm, assessing way, that the lymph nodes in my abdomen and chest wall are not 'causing problems' at the moment. And he says he agrees with Dr Ostler's proposed plan of action: carrying on with Herceptin, but combining it with a new drug called Omnitarg.

∞

Does it make a difference to the outcome, this difference in style? Doctors who make follow-up calls after one has heard bad news? Doctors who are always available by email or mobile phone? Will it make my life longer? I don't know, but I can feel that it makes me more confident, takes some of the fear away.

While I'm getting this attention, thanks entirely to Anthony's client, the best minds in the business are also contacting Peter Ostler, speaking clinical language to a fellow professional – different, I suspect, from the conversations they have with me. This is a process Dr Ostler takes in good part, mostly, becoming irate only once when a French doctor suggests radically departing from my oncologist's already prescribed regime, and there is an outraged yelp of, 'Not a breast specialist is he, he does lungs I think, and what else, kidneys?'

Because – and this is the interesting bit – the treatment options do not vary greatly. Two years ago when this all started I didn't know one cancer doctor from another. I went to my family doctor and did as she said, making an appointment with the first specialist available.

I am treated at Mount Vernon, privately mostly, but it is a local NHS cancer hospital. And on the day I hear my bad news, the reason the 'colleague', David Mills, is in the room is not actually because he's the angel of death, but because he's the man in charge of medical trials – actually, he may be the angel of life.

Omnitarg (Pertuzumab), the drug Dr Ostler puts me on, is a trial drug, which means the only way to get it is to be part of a medical trial – Protocol BO17929, according to the consent form at the end of several pages of information I am given to sign. The form tells me I have read the information – 'version 2.0 date 18 Jan 05' – and that I consent to Roche Products Ltd, makers of the drug, collecting and processing my information, including information about my health, and that, furthermore, if I leave the study, I still consent to this information about me being used.

On 20 June 2006 I sign this document saying, 'I understand that the combination of Herceptin and Omnitarg is an experimental treatment for Metastatic Breast Cancer, and that there are risks of side effects with the drugs.' So far am I from demurring about being involved in a drugs trial, I am already canvassing to be included in a trial for Tykerb (Lapatinib), which is not even available yet in the UK, but about which one of my *Guardian* correspondents, Tina Langson, has emailed me links showing the success Tykerb has had in early trials in the States. 'Yes,' Dr Ostler says, 'if we can get you on Tykerb that will be a good thing. David (Mills) is responsible for it, and he's hoping the drugs company (Glaxo Smith Kline) will be releasing it within a couple of months.'

It is about a week until I fix the names of these drugs into my mind. Neither Anthony nor I can remember them when we drive home, and we can't decipher Dr Ostler's handwriting, though he's written names down for us on a piece of paper. I know the drugs sound like one of Elon's Bionicles, the newest toy in our house, many millions of little pieces which, after following complex 69-page booklets, build up into fighting creatures called Visorak, Hordika, Metro Nui, and Omnitarg. No, Omnitarg's the drug.

But for me, the point is that here at Mount Vernon, the least glitzy of hospitals (looking like a collection of Portakabins actually, and wouldn't be any grander even if you connected all the buildings up following detailed 69-page plans), I'm offered this year's wonder drug, just as – I now know – I'd get at the world's best cancer centres. There is a certain British comfort in that.

18. Cold Comfort

The comfort is short-lived. Weeks into the Omnitarg treatment, and the red lesions on my chest are still growing. It is the hottest of summers, the summer of 2006, and newscasters say things like 'today's heat was record-breaking'. It is the summer of the World Cup.

It could also be the last summer Sara-Jenny spends at home. In September she is leaving for a year's studying in Israel, after which she wants to stay there for university. This is her last year at high school, doing her A levels, legs akimbo on the floor as she spreads her books all around and keeps a tense eye on the footballing gods on the screen.

England go out of the World Cup, the shops are already starting to display winter clothes, and I am facing the usual problem. The sludgy red patches on my skin are growing, and it's too hot to wear any clothes at all, let alone the waistcoat over shirt over sleeveless top that is my mainstay dress code to bulk out the unevenness of being single-breasted. This hot summer Gap comes to the rescue, producing sorbet–coloured lines of sleeveless, thin cotton, that I buy in reams and wear sliced one over the other, the thinness making the heat bearable, the different colours and the layers letting me not look like a freak.

In *Friends* Jennifer Aniston made famous very similar thin cotton tops, designed by C&C California. The Gap ones are a fraction of the price (three for £8 from Gap, rather than a single C&C top at £40), and so I can buy them in the bulk I need. The fineness of the cotton is key: anything harsh irritates the mastectomy area.

'I wonder how many third-world workers have been exploited to make this so cheap,' I say ruefully to my friend Elly, though the thought doesn't stop me buying in bulk.

'I wonder how many women with mastectomies have been exploited by designer companies charging so much for thin cotton tops,' Elly ripostes instantly.

Despairing of ever getting another needle into my now pursed and rigid veins, Peter Ostler has put in a port to dose me with the new drug. This small, round device is placed beneath my skin under local anaesthetic, on the left breast ('How did they get your button inside you, Mummy?' Elon asks, when he sees it, trying it out to see if I will make a funny noise, if I will beep, when he presses it), out of which a tiny tube feeds straight into my veins. Once the bruising from this interesting bit of surgery settles down, and the nurses learn how to puncture the port, it's a much more comfortable way of absorbing intravenous drugs. All good, then, except for one thing: now I look peculiar on both sides, and my emphasis on the clavicle as focal point is becoming ever more perilous. And anyhow, it's just so damn hot.

ತಾ

I travel to the godhead. To Sloan Kettering outpatients' unit on 53rd Street, between Third Avenue and Fourth in New York, an establishment that takes out advertisements in newspapers. One of these ads reads: 'Patients treated at Sloan Kettering often do better than patients treated elsewhere.'

My appointment, at eleven on a Wednesday morning, at this fount of cancer wisdom, is with the mightiest of all the breast-cancer doctors, the one whose name elicits a respectful grunt from all the others. He's called Larry. Larry Norton, MD.

It has taken Anthony's client a matter of minutes to arrange the meeting. The client phones Anthony to say, 'Larry Norton – and you know, Anthony, he is the best – is waiting for Dina's call.'

I phone New York that evening.

'What can I do for you?' The man himself is on the phone, and he's sounding brusque.

'Uh, I was told you're expecting my call,' I say, lamely. Actually I've been told that he's said if I go over to New York he will give me the new wonder drug, Tykerb, in pill form, to bring back with me. So part of me is simply expecting him to say, 'Let me know when you're coming over to pick up a prescription.' It doesn't go quite like that. Far from sounding like he's expecting my call, he doesn't sound like my name means anything to him.

'Are you being harassed on my account?' I say, trying to sound light, and like it doesn't matter to me, I wouldn't dream of bothering him.

'Never mind about that,' he says, in a lightning change of tone. He does this thing of sounding like he's too busy to take in details, but he reacts very quickly to conversational nuances. 'What is it you need?' he asks now.

'Uh, Tykerb?' I say.

'Didn't I speak to you already?' he says. 'When I was in Oxford, I spoke to your doctor, didn't I?' Norton was one of the doctors I spoke to when I first had the news that the cancer had spread. 'These things go through the cracks in my mind, but I spoke to you, didn't I? I don't have any notes for you, though, it's hard for me to remember.'

'Well,' I tell him, 'I'm the one who's had a second recurrence, and I'm now on Omnitarg and Herceptin, but it isn't working.'

'That's right, Omnitarg, I spoke to your doctor, and we decided that was a good plan. I mean, Tykerb's a good drug, but Omnitarg targets more places,' he says. Then, 'I'm speaking to Glaxo Smith Kline (makers of Tykerb) every three or four days. What's happening your end, do you know? Are your doctors making any progress getting hold of it?'

'Um, I don't really know . . . I don't think so. But the point is the Omnitarg isn't working for me,' I say. 'And the thing is, I don't want to get to the next stage . . . I want to stop this at the stage I'm at . . .'

'Not working?' he says, sounding distracted again. 'What do you mean?'

'I can see mine,' I explain. 'I can see the cancer growing. It's on my chest wall, I can see the red patches.'

And now, I have his interest. I can hear a raised alertness in his voice. 'I need to see that,' he says. 'You should come here to be seen, it'll be quick, we'll have you in and out, but we can register you as a patient, and then I'll have your notes in front of me.'

And then he says, very definitely, 'I have something here that will be absolutely right for you, a drug we're working on, it's called 17AAG, but you have to come here to get it. It's only available at Memorial (Sloan Kettering). We're using it with Herceptin and we're having very good results, including one complete remission.'

The day after this phone conversation I go to Mount Vernon for another round of combined Herceptin/Omnitarg treatment, a drug combination I am given once every three weeks. It's a three-day process: on the Wednesday I go for an echo, a scan that monitors my heart, then on the Thursday there is the trial-required blood test, and on the Friday, the infusion of Herceptin, followed by Omnitarg. In with that mix I also fit in a teddy bears' picnic at Elon's school, but Anthony has to stand in for me at the special end-of-term assembly where mothers who have helped out during the year are specially thanked. In a stifling school hall, where all the speeches go on far too long, Anthony accepts a small round glass plate from Elon on my behalf, while I sit in a light-filled hospital ward, looking out on Mount Vernon's green spaces, and discuss my Larry Norton conversation with Peter Ostler.

'You should go to New York,' he says at once. He is, in his quiet way, completely unequivocal. He says he hasn't heard of 17AAG, though he looks it up after we speak. 'It's nothing we're even working on here yet,' he says, later.

These hours in hospital wards are like time removed from normal life. You have to be there, and you can't do anything other than receive drugs through the drip. It is because Omnitarg is a trial drug and therefore given through the NHS that I am in a regular ward, a room with eight beds, no bedside phone lines or televisions, unlike paid-for, 'private' hospital rooms. If you want privacy in these rooms, you draw a curtain round your bed, which shuts you in, but still means every word can be heard by all the other patients and their visitors. There are long stretches of silence, people muted by the experience they're living through, sitting with their hands in their laps. In these wards, the nurses decide when the overhead lights come on and go off, and the evening meal is brought round at five in the afternoon, a time when the smallest children eat.

'Shake me and I'll rattle,' one woman says to a nurse handing her some more pills. I am, always, the youngest in this cancer ward; everybody is asked their date of birth as a protocol before the drugs are dispensed, and so I hear the answers: '1929' or '1935'. When I try to use my phone, to answer calls and also book my plane ticket to New York next week, an officious nurse loudly places a notice next to my head: MOBILE PHONES MUST BE SWITCHED OFF, AS THEY INTERFERE WITH THE EQUIPMENT.

In the bed next to mine, a woman is preparing to leave this ward, the Marie Curie ward, to move to a hospice. She talks about how she's known her husband since they were both five years old, how they went to the same playgroup, lived in streets five minutes away from each other. He sits next to her, unmoving, not speaking. 'Are you just going to sit there all day?' she snaps at him, at one point. 'I'm getting both barrels,' the husband tells the doctor, later.

There is companionship on NHS wards, but there is no privacy. Across from me a woman is dying, I think. Her Indian relatives are keening and praying around her insistently, a noise so low it takes a while to realize what it is. Everybody on the ward can hear when a junior doctor comes in and tells the woman's male relatives that the consultants have decided she is unable to take any more chemotherapy. I feel incredibly angry that the consultant hasn't come to give her this news himself, and I feel deeply embarrassed when Dr Ostler, my consultant, comes back to see me twice.

And there is war, in Israel. Marganit and Chloë are both away now, on summer camps touring Israel. The camps don't allow mobile phones; Marganit is the only child who has managed to keep hers, and she phones home regularly. The war is in the north, on the border with Lebanon, so all the youth touring Israel this summer are being kept in the south, living on kibbutzim and sleeping on beaches in Eilat. There is a different sense of time when you are at camp too: the first few days go slowly, can be difficult, and then the weeks fly by.

In our house, the days of this war are lines etched on Anthony's face. Max, his oldest child, his twenty-four-year-old son, is doing army service in Israel, and his unit is posted in the north, where the fighting is. On Sunday, the day before I am due to fly to New York, there is a feature piece in the *Sunday Times* about the lives of the Israeli soldiers who are in the middle of the combat. The piece is structured round the story of a Jewish boy from England, whose father is an eminent lawyer, and who is fielding texts from his parents asking how he is. It is Max, and the phone starts ringing early Sunday morning, before Max can get through to either of his parents to say he has been quoted in the paper. Max texts home most days – texts two homes, his mother and his father – saying, 'I'm fine, and I'm eating.' But the newspaper article says he looks pale and tired.

That Sunday afternoon there is a peace rally, a demonstration of support by the Jewish community for Israel, to which we all go, and then on Monday I leave for New York. On the plane, there is the 24-page fax to wade through from Sloan Kettering. It announces, in a quite daunting way, that I am bidden to turn up 'one and one half hours prior to the appointment'. I have to register at the international centre, a process which does indeed take the full hour and a half, and culminates in the handing over of a $3000 deposit. No small sum. 'In the UK,' I tell the extremely nice, and not at all daunting, woman who takes me through the registration process, 'you just turn up, and you get your medical treatment.'

'I know, I know,' she says, 'in my country too, but here it is all about papers and forms.'

There are forms telling me about my rights to privacy, and Sloan Kettering's rights to my tissues and body samples. Then there's the form that explains when they can sue me, and when I can sue them.

I finally meet Larry Norton at 12.15. Just a disembodied voice at first, apologizing from halfway down the corridor. 'I'm sorry, sorry, sorry – sorry you've been kept waiting.' And in he comes, short, thinning grey hair, beaming and quizzical-looking, quite like the Cheshire cat actually, a similarity reinforced over the next hour when he keeps springing up from his chair, bobbing in and out of the room, disappearing and reappearing.

'Yes,' he says, looking at me appraisingly, 'I'm glad you came over. I'm really good, but I can't do this on the phone.' And then he adds, 'Really sorry about the wait, normally Wednesday isn't my clinic day; I get caught up with all this administration.' And then later: 'I'm going to spend a lot of time with you, you came all the way over here to see me.'

I can't imagine an English doctor ever using that phrase – 'I'm really good' – let alone employing Norton's tone of matter-of-factness. And no English doctor would do this either: when Norton examines the lesions on my chest, when he first sees me sitting stripped to the waist on the hospital bed in the consulting room, he says, in the most paternal of ways, 'Come on, now, sit up straight,' like I'm a candidate for *America's Next Top Model* and he's my coach to success. It's a New York emphasis on posture and making the absolute best of oneself.

He does share one quality with the doctors who have been treating me throughout this illness. Larry Norton could not be more different in manner and bearing from Mr Al-Dubaisi but they both react in exactly the same way to something I tell them as they take an initial history from me. All that time ago, more than two years now, when I first met Mr Al-Dubaisi, he wasn't going to allow me a second's guilt or anxiety over the fact that I came to him with a lump that had grown big on my watch.

And now, when Larry Norton asks me about the lump and first having it diagnosed, and I say to him, 'Diagnosed June 2004, but I'd been aware of it for much longer, probably three years or so,' I see him swiftly lower his face so I won't be affected by his expression. And what was the reaction that crossed his face? Sheer regret, as clear as if it was his own illness, and just that. They have the complete range of personality defects, these doctors in whom I place my life and trust, but every single time I am pierced through by this single fact: they really care.

'Where is Mount Vernon Cancer Hospital?' he asks, changing the subject, looking up from the sheaf of referral notes.

'Uh, North London,' I say.

'Yes, but where, where exactly?' My mind has gone completely blank, I can't remember the name of the area Mount Vernon is in – any minute now he's going to start thinking I've just made the whole cancer story up. But while I'm floundering, he offers the classic New Yorker's take on London: 'In relation to Harrods,' he says, 'where is it in relation to Harrods?'

Norton calls in a woman colleague to take a look at the red marks surrounding the scar on my chest. These marks, it seems to me, are what interest the doctors and later, when I am fully clothed again, and we're once more sitting on opposite sides of a pale wooden desk, I ask him what the fascination is.

'What is it about the red marks?' I ask, and he looks a little taken aback. 'Because I could hear it in your voice over the phone as well, when I said to you that I can see my cancer, can see it growing, and that's when you said, "You need to come over here, I need to see that."'

He answers the question straight on. 'Yes,' he says, 'exactly that, because we can see it.' And then he gives the American spin: 'Just as you can see it growing, we'll be able to see it getting smaller when you start here with us.'

He does one of his disappearing tricks and his colleague, the woman doctor, sits on a desk and chats to me. 'Obviously,' I say to her, 'if it's a difference between life and death, then of course we'll move to New York, but if it isn't . . . well, there's several children involved, it's a big disruption.'

'I wouldn't like to say it's life and death,' she says, 'it's not as clear-cut as that.' She tells me they have seventeen patients on 17AAG and, of those, seven have responded to the drug to some extent, including the one woman who is in near-complete remission.

'And the other ten?' I ask. She shakes her head – no, nothing.

Norton's certain tone begins to fade. When he comes back into the room, and I repeat the news that there are several children involved in this potential move to the States, he says, 'Ah,' and makes little marks on the lined paper in front of him.

Back out on the hot midday, dog-end of summer New York city streets, where the Fifth Avenue shop windows are displaying mannequins in autumn clothes, the red rash that's been creeping up my skin for a few days now becomes unbearable. When I showed it to Norton he said, 'Yes, of course, classic EGFH skin symptom.' Omnitarg is a drug that targets epidermal growth factor, hence the abbreviation, basically blocking the cancer cells from growing.

'So can you give me something to help?' I ask Norton.

'We'll take you off the Omnitarg,' he said, 'that's what we'll do.' He and his colleague tell me that 17AAG has hardly any side effects. As far as they know, it's not bad for the heart, and doesn't cause skin rashes, nausea, or hair to fall out. 'Fatigue,' the woman doctor says, 'that's it, really.' What kind of fatigue? 'Well,' she says, 'you haven't had much chemo, really, but it's the kind of fatigue our patients on chemotherapy report. My sense is it affects different people differently.'

'My sense,' I say, 'is that having small children is very effective. Because they don't let you sleep . . .'

∾

If I have any jet lag it's indistinguishable from the cancer or cancer-treatment fatigue I've lived with for too long now, so after the two-day jaunt to New York it's straight to Mount Vernon, that hospital situated in an outer part of London near Watford, having yet another CT scan to see what effect, if any, the Omnitarg is having.

I'm craning down to look at the red patches on my chest, and saying, 'There's some white there, can you see? Looks like it's clearing a bit, unless that's some new kind of cancer . . .' I put in quickly, just so I can cover all the options before I look foolish, like I live under too many illusions, too hopeful, not hard-bitten enough.

'Uh, no,' Dr Ostler's research assistant, Jenny, says to me, just covering her surprise that I haven't realized.

'That's not cancer, that's your normal tissue, your normal skin, showing through.' So the white area that has opened up in the spreading red triangle is my old skin, my healthy untumoured, undamaged skin cells putting in a reappearance. The reversal of cancer, then? Well, not to be too journalistic about this, not doing that declaiming headlines thing, talking about cures, we can call this something of a reverse, or as the doctors put it, 'stable disease'.

A bit later on, Peter Ostler says, a little wryly under the barrage of questions from Anthony and me: 'Look, this is a good-news consultation, not a bad-news one.'

It takes a while for good news to sink in, I guess. About as long as the bad news, really. It's two years and three months since I first learned that I have breast cancer. And I'm still waiting for it to go away, still thinking, OK, I've done this now, I'm ready for the aftershock to set in, you know, the delayed reaction you get when the threat's gone away. Delayed because you've been using every resource to just carry on normally with the executioners at the gates. I haven't yet realized that I *have* cancer; I keep thinking it's something I caught, have dealt with now, and so it's time for it to be in the past.

But with the realization that no, it's something I have now, for ever, really, comes the good news. This, what I'm experiencing, is what they mean when they talk about 'living with cancer', as opposed to dying from it. Or that's the hope, anyhow. That the drugs in the armoury are effective enough, and plenteous enough, to keep cancers under control. It isn't going away – it's not ever going to go away, Dr Ostler makes a point of repeating to me, cautiously, during most consultations – but we can now say it's under control. Somewhat under control, anyhow. For the moment.

I'm on my fifth round of Herceptin combined with Omnitarg. I'm the first person Dr Ostler – clinical director of Mount Vernon Cancer Hospital, head of some fifteen clinical oncologists, three medical oncologists, two consultant haematologists and assorted research fellows – has ever treated with Omnitarg.

I can't say how much Omnitarg costs; it's only available as a trial drug, and hasn't been given a price yet. These are the outer reaches of cancer treatment. It takes about an hour to administer. So far, I've fallen asleep each time, for about forty minutes, after the drip is finished. Fallen asleep in a way that is unusual for me, absolutely unable to stay awake. But that could be because I'm having it in a ward which tends to be overheated and, because the Herceptin goes in first over ninety minutes, followed by the Omnitarg, maybe I'm just drowsy from lying around in a hospital bed for hours.

There's a lurking exhaustion round the edges of my consciousness. But is that the drugs? Who knows? The point about these drugs – Omnitarg, 17AAG, Tykerb (Lapatinib) – is their side effects are not brutal, they are comfortably lived with – well, out here, in the furthest reaches of cancer treatment. And the point about cancer treatment today seems to be that the doctors give you a drug, it works for a while, then – like bugs and antibiotics – the cancer grows resistant, so they need another drug to try out for some more years.

The most hopeful of the new drugs appears to be

Tykerb, but all the doctors across the world are waiting for the drugs company to release it. Every time I hear it discussed, it's 'in another few weeks'. In the meantime Larry Norton emails Peter Ostler to say that Professor Ian Judson at the Royal Marsden is working with 17AAG right here in the UK, after all, and I should go to see him.

I phone Professor Judson and, unusually, he answers the phone himself with a soft 'hello'. I'm so surprised I don't say anything for a moment, and he says, 'Ian Judson here.'

'Oh,' I say, 'I need to make an appointment.'

'Fine,' he replies, 'let me see which secretary to put you through to – uh, clinical, no I'll put you through to my PA.'

'You have half a dozen secretaries and you still answer the phone yourself, that's great,' I say.

In the event it's his colleague, a Dr de Bono, who talks to me about 17AAG. Well, 17 Dmeg, in fact, a newer version of the drug, since the original one made patients 'smell'. I leave home at six in the morning for this appointment at the Royal Marsden in Sutton, Surrey. I can take one train to get there, an hour's jaunt, and a five-minute ride in a taxi. At reception they give you forms asking if it's all right for them to use your tissues for research. Meanwhile, ladies in aprons are setting up tables, selling gifts and books to raise money for the hospital.

A short wait and I'm called in to a small yellow-painted cubicle. 'Doctor will be with you as and when . . .' the research assistant says, halfway out of the room before she's finished her sentence. This is NHS-style patient treatment, none of the niceties of the private hospitals, the offers of tea and biscuits.

I wait about another ten minutes before another research assistant appears, a young woman with long black hair and a pale pink jumper. I have time to study exactly what she's wearing because her English is so heavily accented I can't understand most of it. She's Italian, though she's working at a hospital in Switzerland, but is here for six months. My English is acutely tuned, I'd say, but I can't make out every third word she says, so I keep asking her to repeat words like 'observations' and 'trial slots'. It makes me wonder how somebody whose own native language isn't English would cope.

I ask her lots of questions, all with a second assistant listening. This other researcher is from Poland and came here fourteen years ago. 'Oh,' I say, 'you must have been one of the first wave of Polish immigrants then?'

'Not really,' she answers, shaking her head with a wry smile, like she's telling me I know as little about her immigrant's experience as my impatience implies she understands too little about how it is to have cancer. The communication gap between us three is now so huge the two women call in the consultant. 'He will answer your questions,' they say, and leave hurriedly, and happily.

Dr de Bono is a little guy, with not much hair. I'm trying hard to get a physical sense of him, because on the train here I've been reading John Updike, and his descriptions of people's appearances are so accurate you can smell them. But the Updike magic isn't catching and the only image I can summon is that of a ping-pong ball when the doctor bounces in.

And then, once he starts talking, all I get is an incredibly battered feeling, and I leave in tears, out into pouring, sleeting rain. He says things that frighten me, about the drugs only working for a matter of months, and then, 'You're not a scientist, are you?' He doesn't mean it to sound harsh, he's wrestling with his own sense of this cancer. He says it is guesswork as to which drugs will work. The doctors try different combinations of drugs and hope that one will control the tumour growth.

'I feel like I'm in a dark room,' I tell him, 'and you're all chucking apples at me, hoping one will hit home.'

Yes, he admits, as other doctors have explained to me before. The problem is, every cancer is different, every tumour is different. But that is only one part of the problem. The real difficulty is an economic one.

'It's commercial,' Dr de Bono says. 'The drugs companies won't put money into diagnosing the structures of tumours, only into cures. We did it here, worked out a test for Her-2 – but that wasn't until five years after Herceptin was developed.' You can make a profit, you see, out of 'curing' people; they pay for the medicine. Work out the cause, though, and they may not need the medicine after all.

I am crying uncontrollably when I leave the Marsden and phone Anthony. 'I shouldn't have come on my own,' I weep, adding, 'that's it with the second opinions; I just want to speak to the doctors I know from now on.'

Meanwhile, I have a book deadline. Engaging in deeply complicated diversionary tactics, I take a break from not thinking about the book deadline to canvas some endorsements for the book cover (cover, not content, see?). Philip Pullman, author of the *His Dark Materials* trilogy, a children's author whose fame is second only to J. K. Rowling, and who emailed me to wish me well the day the first of my *Guardian* pieces about this illness was printed, and Cherie Blair, another email respondent to my newspaper columns, both immediately offer their support. Cherie Blair, maternal, tells me not to worry about the encroaching deadline and how many more words I have to go, but 'think how far you've come'.

The deadline is imminent, and the publishers say 'early delivery would be appreciated'. So that's no consideration at all given to the spate of Jewish holidays about to break over us. We are in the season of apple and honey, Rosh Hashana, followed by Yom Kippur, and then, the one most haven't heard about, Succot, where Orthodox Jews build wooden structures outside their houses and eat and study outside for seven days (in warm coats and wellingtons, usually, in this country). Anthony's son Max will be home for a month. Because he is a *chayal boded* – a soldier whose family are abroad – he is given a very long leave. And Sara-Jenny, happily settled in Israel, is coming back for a ten-day visit. It is the season of apples and honey.

Epilogue

I am on the phone to my eldest sister, Tovit, ten years older than me. 'How did you not know about Bubbe Pesha?' she asks me, talking about our grandmother who died of breast cancer. 'It's as if you grew up in a different home from the one I lived in. All my life I knew about her being ill, there were all the phone calls, back and forth. I've been having mammograms for years.'

I tell her I remember when Bubbe Pesha died, and my mother flew off to America in the middle of the night. Before she went, she said goodbye to me on the stairs, and that 'Bubbe Pesha loved you, you know'.

I remember my grandmother, a kind woman who always had a walking frame to lean on – when I knew her anyhow – and had leather-bound copies of Charles Dickens books in her house, which I read in the room full of heavy furniture where I slept when I stayed there.

Tovit says, 'I must have been five when she had her operation (the mastectomy, she means). I remember being in her room once and her sadness at the operation, and I thought, what's the fuss about, it's not like it's an arm or a leg.'

I hear echoes of Anne Fine when Tovit tells me this, and I say that I think that's quite an astute point for a five-year-old. But my older sister won't countenance that, insists it was a heartless, childish comment and berates herself for it.

She tells me my grandmother tried every drug, every cure available to her, including some potion called 'rifuin' developed by a Rabbi Tendler. My grandmother lived thirteen years after her mastectomy.

There's a conversation I have with Peter Ostler these days. I say, 'Am I going to live any longer if I take these drugs, or am I just using up whole days of what life I have left, trekking backwards and forwards to hospital for treatment and scans and heart monitoring? Maybe I'd live just as long and just as well without anything.'

He replies that when the disadvantages outweigh the benefits then he becomes a 'nihilist', an advocate of doing nothing, but that if I stopped taking the drugs now he thinks I'd become much more ill much more quickly. But he and his colleagues both have patients who just stop coming for treatment after a while. 'Why?' I ask. He *shrugs his shoulders.*

David Mills says he has a patient with lesions on her chest – like mine, though I call them red patches – and this woman has stopped taking all medication. Her lesions 'come and go', he says. He doesn't know why, 'maybe it's her own antibodies coming into play'. At the Royal Marsden, Dr de Bono tells me he had a patient whose lesions cleared completely, but the cancer came back anyhow, internally, and she died within three years.

The doctors call this the 'realm of the experimental'.

We're on the outer edges of cancer treatment here, they say, too often for my liking.

∞

In the back of my car, Elon and a friend from school are having a conversation. I'm obsessing about drugs, and whether I'm taking enough control of my treatment, so I miss the first bits of their chatter, fading back in only when I hear Elon saying, 'What's that, bosoms?'

'These,' the six-year-old, worldly girlfriend replies, clutching her chest. 'Women have huge ones, boys only have tiny ones. When I'm older, I'm going to have really big ones.'

'Oh, you mean where babies have food from?' Elon says. My baby, my boy that I was so worried about wresting from the breast, is truly on steak and chips now.

'I just don't know how they can do it,' Elon is saying, some disgust in his voice. 'You know, that means they are giving the babies the food from their own bodies, with all their germs and everything.'

He pauses a moment, the full horror of the unhygienic scenario sinking in, then carries on perfectly matter-of-factly, to say, 'My mum has e-e-e-norrrr-mous ones.'

I am tuned right in to their conversation now, so I am quite sure he uses the plural 'ones' not the singular 'one' and he does this without any self-consciousness at all, absolutely no inflection of any doubt in his voice. And as the two children collapse into giggles, Elon's relish at the word 'enormous' fills the car.